Women and distance learning: Approaches to study and the learning experience

Dedication

This book is dedicated to my mother, Mina Downey, who gave me the inspiration to study.

Women and distance learning: Approaches to study and the learning experience

by

Ros Carnwell

APS Publishing
The Old School, Tollard Royal, Salisbury, Wiltshire, SP5 5PW
www.apspublishing.co.uk

British Library Cataloguing in Publication Data
A catalogue record for this book is available from the British Library

ISBN 0 9537234 6 1

Printed in the UK by Selwood Printing Ltd, Burgess Hill

Contents

Acknowledgements

I would like to acknowledge the following people, without whose help and support this book would not have reached fruition. First, the students who readily gave of their time to be interviewed or complete questionnaires; secondly, my research supervisor, Neil Moreland, who provided advice on the development of the original research; thirdly, the University of Wolverhampton, for allowing me to conduct the research; and, finally, to my husband, Keith, for his enduring patience and support.

Preface

Distance learning has become increasingly popular as a mode of learning. Its use is likely to increase still further with the promise of e-universities and corresponding developments in technology-mediated learning. The pace of change is fast and is determined largely by technological innovation and globalisation. Such changes do not always take account of the individual needs of students, the dominant ideology being, to deliver high quality learning as efficiently as possible. While these changes are taking place, women are still grappling with the problems of finding time to study and coping with the family and work commitments. This book is based on the premise that delivery of distance learning, both paper-based materials and technologically-mediated, fails to take into account students' individual learning needs. Such needs often arise from the way in which students approach their study, and, although there is a wealth of research into learning style, strategies and approaches to study, these are rarely reflected adequately in learning materials or support services available. Technological advances that make assumptions about women's access to computers, and their ability to make adequate use of them, will further compound this lack of provision.

This book attempts to address this imbalance by focussing on the approaches to study of women distance learners, and the impact these approaches have on other factors, such as curriculum design, the role of the tutor, learning support needs, and coping strategies. The book is based on in-depth interviews of twenty women distance learners. *Chapter 1* discusses the nature of distance learning and is followed by a review of literature covering learning styles, strategies, approaches to study and learning preferences, in *Chapter 2*. In *Chapters 3* and *4*, the research into the approaches to study of the twenty participants, and the impact of these approaches for delivery of distance learning, is explained. *Chapter 5* explores the findings of the research by focussing on coping strategies used by women distance learners, and *Chapter 6* concludes the text by inviting readers to reflect on the content of the book in relation to their own experiences of learning and learning needs. This personal reflection is a feature throughout the book and is consistent with the distance learning philosophy. The book also reflects my personal experience of being a distance learning student and distance learning tutor for many years.

Ros Carnwell: 2001

1
Distance learning and opportunities for women learners

Introduction

Distance learning has become increasingly popular as a mode of study. It is common throughout many disciplines, including business administration and the health professions, such as nursing, medicine and professions allied to medicine. Since the research on which this book is based involved nurses, the background to distance learning in nursing will first be briefly outlined. As all the nurses interviewed for this research were women, however, the book does not focus on distance learning in *nursing*, but on *women* as distance learners.

The use of distance learning in nursing gained prominence during the 1980s, when it was used primarily to facilitate the conversion of enrolled nurses to registered nurse status. Later, as specialist practitioner roles developed (United Kingdom Central Council for Nursing, Midwifery, and Health Visiting: UKCC, 1994), the need for traditionally qualified nurses to gain diploma status also increased. Many nurses achieved this through studying English National Board (ENB) courses, but, for others, release from duties combined with competing family commitments proved difficult. In this respect, female nurses may have much in common with other women distance learners who wish to develop, or even change a career, by studying at a distance. During the 1990s, distance learning programmes in various higher education institutions responded to this challenge, and now distance learning programmes for qualified nurses are a common mode of study. This chapter will explore the nature and philosophy of distance learning and its use in providing learning opportunities for women.

The chapter is divided into five sections. First, characteristics of distance learning are explored, including its advantages and limitations. This is followed by a comparison between distance learning and campus-based study. These distinctions have important implications for the role of the tutor and, therefore, a section is devoted to the role of the tutor in distance learning. Sections on women as distance learners and distance learning opportunities for women conclude the chapter.

Characteristics of distance learning

What is distance learning and how does it differ from open learning? For those who enrol on a distance learning programme of study, what can they realistically expect? Distance learning can be defined as learning that takes place geographically separate from the institution at which the student is registered. It is for this very reason that distance learning has become increasingly popular for women who wish to gain academic credit, without physically attending the institution with which they are registered. Keegan (1980) develops this further, suggesting that distance learning has the following characteristics:

- separation of teacher and learner
- the use of media for instructional purposes
- opportunity for dialogue between the learner, the text materials and tutors
- the possibility of occasional meetings.

Technology has advanced since Keegan suggested these characteristics in 1980, and distance learning materials are often available on the World Wide Web and delivered through video conferencing. Other characteristics suggested by Keegan remain equally valid, despite these new methods of delivery. Conversations between students and tutors are crucial in enabling students to understand learning materials, whether they are in text or computerised form. These conversations may take place by telephone, or through more formal group tutorials.

Although the terms 'distance learning' and 'open learning' are often used interchangeably, the two methods of delivery are distinct. Open learning is so defined because it is openly accessible and, therefore, not constrained by usual entry requirements. Open learning can be classroom-based, although open/distance learning materials are often used as a learning resource. The Open University is a typical example of 'open' learning. Open University courses are accessible to all, regardless of formal qualifications, distance learning materials are used, and class-based group tutorials are common. This book is about *distance learning*, however, and having dispensed with these important distinctions, this chapter will now consider the main advantages and disadvantages of distance learning for women who wish to engage in further study.

During the 1970s and 1980s numerous authors, including Wedemeyer (1977), Keegan (1985), Holmberg (1989) and Rumble (1989), identified several advantages of distance learning. These advantages included: flexibility, allowing students to begin and finish courses and submit assignments as they wish; and autonomy and freedom for students to pursue their own learning goals (see *Table 1.1*). In addition to these generally agreed advantages, Rogers (1986) proposes that distance learning materials present information in varied forms that draw on life experiences, thereby arousing emotional responses, which may occur in private. She suggests that this process facilitates 'mindful' acquisition through actively engaging students, allowing both in-depth study, as well as broader analysis of certain issues.

In comparing these advantages with the limitations of distance learning (see *Table 1.1*), some authors argue that distance learning materials 'commodify' knowledge, thereby perpetuating the social philosophies of those who control it (Chesterton, 1985). According to Tait (1988: 98), this reflects:

> *'a hierarchical image of society in which authority and power reside with those who are the holders and regulators of expert knowledge'.*

Snell *et al* (1987) further argue that this control over knowledge, combined with depersonalisation of the teacher role, make it more difficult for students to question the value given to knowledge and gain power over it.

This concern with students gaining power over knowledge is reflected in other criticisms of distance learning in relation to the design of the materials. Such criticisms include: the encouragement of rote learning, due to the requirement to regurgitate materials for assignments (Perraton, 1983), and subordination of individual students' learning needs to the package itself, so that the student becomes a passive consumer of knowledge (Harris, 1976; Sewart, 1987). So, distance learning can either be viewed as a flexible learning opportunity in which students can be genuinely autonomous, or as a method of learning in which knowledge becomes a commodity that is controlled by those who have power over it.

Table 1.1: Advantages and limitations of distance learning

Advantages	Limitations
Flexibility, allowing students to begin and finish courses and submit assignments as they wish	Control of knowledge by material writers—knowledge as a commodity
Autonomy	Knowledge as a commodity makes it more difficult for students to gain power over it
Freedom for students to pursue their own learning goals	Regurgitation of learning materials causes 'rote learning'
Active engagement in in-depth study fosters 'mindful' acquisition of knowledge, and application to real life experiences	Subordination of the needs of students to the learning package, so that students becomes passive consumers of commodity of knowledge

The advantages listed in *Table 1.1* need to be treated with some caution, due to variations in distance learning provision. Some programmes, for example, allow students to enrol on a course of study at whatever point in the academic year they wish, while others impose minor restrictions, with several enrolment points per year. Likewise, in some programmes, students may submit their assignments whenever they wish, although annual examination boards often impose restrictions. It is often the case that students who enrol early in the academic year have a longer period to produce their assignment. By contrast, enrolment during the early summer often results in accelerated learning for those wishing to access an advanced programme of study in the autumn term, for which the distance learning course is a prerequisite. It is worth finding out, when deciding to embark on a distance learning programme, what the requirements are for enrolment and submission of assignments.

As indicated in *Table 1.1*, being autonomous in learning is certainly one of the main advantages of distance learning and includes the ability to determine one's own pace, place and time of learning. Freedom to pursue one's own learning goals is an advantage, although goals will always be determined too, by the learning outcomes imposed by the programme of study. This is particularly so in professional courses that are validated by external bodies.

The limitations identified in *Table 1.1* raise important issues that have been challenged by several authors. Evans and Nation (1989) argue, for example, that regardless of the 'packaging' of materials, students will devise their own way of working through them. Students are not as easily manipulated, therefore, as course writers seem to imagine (Gibbs *et al*, 1982), and are quite capable of gaining power of learning materials. As will be seen in *Chapter 2*, students adopt different learning styles, approaches to study, and learning strategies when using distance learning materials.

Comparing distance learning with class-based study

One way of clarifying what can be expected from distance learning, is to compare distance learning with class-based study (see *Table 1.2*). It has already been suggested that, in distance learning, the needs of individual students are subordinated to the needs of the package. In class-based study the needs of individual students are also subordinated, but to the needs of the whole group (Stewart, 1985). Moreover, students' need for feedback is often met more successfully in distance learning, as assignment feedback is a crucial means of communicating with students. Tutors often anticipate a student's response to a particular script comment and then respond to it in their assignment feedback. By comparison, class-based students rely on peers, as well as tutors, for feedback and, later, assignment feedback can be supported by further discussion, if students take up opportunities offered. Cropley and Kahl

(1983) consider psychological characteristics in relation to both distance education and face-to-face learning. They propose six 'core dimensions' of teaching/learning situations that comprise: organisation of learning; motivation; learning processes; communication processes; didactic activities and materials; and evaluation and feedback. These dimensions are incorporated into *Table 1.2*.

Table 1.2: A comparison of distance learning and class-based study

	Distance learning	Class-based study
Individual student needs	Subordinated to package	Subordinated to needs of whole class
Reassurance about performance	Relies on personal feedback from tutor	Compares self with peers in the group
Organisation of learning	Determined by student	Determined by tutor—may be too fast or too slow
Motivation	Requires internal motivation due to influence of situations in which behaviours, not associated with study, are usual	More natural in situations where the natural thing to do is learn
Learning processes	Balance learning with other competing demands on time. Assignment preparation has equal value to reading learning materials	Competing demands on time may encroach on reading, assignment completion etc., with students believing that the only learning of value is that which occurs in the classroom
Communication processes	Less opportunity to use the teacher as a role model or to learn by identification with the values and beliefs of the teacher	Moment by moment student feedback and non-verbal communication may affect the communication process in either a positive or negative way
Didactic activities and materials	Well-organised and clear, but impersonal and rigid	More personal and responsive to students' needs
Evaluation and feedback	Students have more control over what to send in for evaluation, therefore, greater exploration, autonomy, and independence	Evaluation partly measures the ability to fit into the organisation's goals

Whether or not internal motivation will generate more effective learning is debatable and it is arguable that motivation comes naturally in a classroom setting—numerous other psycho-social factors must surely be at work, such as competing demands on time and interest in the subject.

What is clear from the characteristics of distance learning, as it compares to class-based learning, is that it requires a good deal of autonomy on the part of the student. By autonomy is meant the ability of learners to accept responsibility for, and to self-manage, their own learning (Chene, 1983). According to Chene, this relies not only on the will to learn, but also on an awareness of the learning process and the ability to make critical judgements (Chene, 1983). As indicated in *Table 1.2*, the role of the tutor differs considerably between distance learning and class-based study. In distance learning, for example, the tutor is far less visible and this fact alone is likely to have a bearing on student autonomy. Students accepting responsibility for their own learning, however, does not mean that tutors abdicate responsibility for facilitating learning. Rather, the role of the tutor takes on a different form and this needs to be considered when selecting a distance learning programme of study.

The role of the tutor in distance education

Tutors have the important role of mediating between students' needs and the requirements of the course team (Naylor *et al*, 1990), good tutoring being as important as well-designed packages in producing good quality learning (Bailey, 1992). Thus, although learning packages will be designed in such a way as to ensure that learning outcomes can be achieved, the tutor is crucial in enabling students to make the best use of the learning experience. For distance education tutors, the fact that content is contained within course materials, frees their time to become 'a genuine, respecting, open person first and a content expert second' (Burge, 1988: 15). The distance education tutor is, therefore, a facilitator of information rather than a communicator of information.

However, the facilitator role creates a dilemma for distance education tutors and students alike. Tutors often remain unsure of how much to intervene in students' learning. A balance is needed between offering too much support and advice, and leaving students to fight for survival (Holmberg, 1989). As Holmberg points out, this is aggravated by the additional family and social commitments involved with being adult students. For women working full-time while continuing their studies, this balance is particularly important and students need to be prepared to negotiate their support needs with tutors.

Bailey (1992) has examined the role of the tutor as a facilitator in open learning. She argues that the locus of control should pass to the students who should take responsibility for self-assessment, diagnosing strengths and weakness, formulating study plans and using feedback. Bailey acknowledges, however, that this may be impeded by the more authoritarian models of learning inherited by both students and tutors. Tutors vary widely in their need for power and control, some knowing no other style for working with learners (Burge, 1988). Other tutors may lack confidence in self-direction and compensate by packing the course with taught theory (Leonard and Jowett, 1990). Indeed, Cunningham (1987) suggests that, when faced with students who have specific learning difficulties, tutors are most likely to resort to teaching the students about the subject, and teaching study skills (e.g. essay writing). Cunningham advocated, instead, the identification of unsuccessful patterns in the student's learning and to change the pattern rather than 'try harder'. This may include examining triggers or negative anchors that act as precursors to learning patterns, or enabling students to change their internal mental map of how they learn by reframing confusions to include the possibility of learning.

According to Bailey, the learning context should shift from focussing on static elements of knowledge towards the learning process itself. Thus, the essential roles of the tutor include: counselling, trouble-shooting and helping learners manage their learning (Bailey, 1992). This process should help students to fit new knowledge contained in packages into their own pre-existing intellectual framework, as well as their everyday attitudes and behaviour (Sewart, 1987: 32). Thus, in facilitating distance learners, educators need to *know* their students and, as Diaz and Cartnal (1999) suggest, this might involve assessing the learning styles of students when they enrol. Support and guidance can then be adapted to suit individual learning needs, as will be discussed further in *Chapter 4*.

The role of the tutor is important in sustaining the autonomous and empowering nature of distance learning.These characteristics are emancipating for students, and this factor has captured the hearts and minds of women learners. This opening chapter would not be complete, therefore, without a consideration of women as distance learners.

Women as distance learners

Whether or not they are employed, women still carry the main burden of domestic responsibility (Pym, 1992). Moreover, homemaking demands are not reduced when a woman becomes a mature learner (Green, 1987). According to von Prummer and Rossie (1988), the assumptions surrounding the stress involved in combining paid, unpaid work, and study is contradicted by the fact that distance education is considered particularly suited to women who are housebound, since absence from home is not required.

Pym and Atkinson (1990) found that only 4% of survey respondents anticipated no emotional support from family and friends, with 9% expecting no practical support. Pym (1992) further suggests that, although there is no quantitative evidence, experience indicates that many women are surprised, grieved, and puzzled by the lack of support they receive. Pym (1992: 386) goes on to suggest that:

> *'... husbands fear that a wife may change as a result of further education, and that he may be 'left behind' or may lose his authority within the family'.*

Women have also been found to feel more isolated in their studies than men feel. Even when data was controlled for employment and household type, women in employment were more likely than men to feel that their isolation was a problem (Kirkup and von Prummer, 1990).

It could be that the isolation and lack of support experienced by women, results in a need to learn collaboratively. Von Prummer and Rossie (1988) stress that women have a greater preference than men for learning in the company of others, and sharing their problems and progress. It would appear, therefore, that, although women would gain more from tutorials than men, they have less opportunity to attend. Despite this, von Prummer and Rossie (1988) found that more women than men attended a study centre during their first year of study. Kirkup and von Prummer (1990) found similar gender characteristics in a large survey of over 2,000 students in the UK and German Open Universities. They also comment on the desire of women for interactive learning and study centre attendance. In both the German and UK Open Universities women made greater efforts to overcome problems of distance and accessibility in order to attend study centres.

Specific difficulties experienced by women in relation to attending tutorials centred on transport difficulties, personal safety, and the combined pressures of work and family commitments (Kirkup and von Prummer, 1990). Men's attendance was also affected by pressures of work, but, rather than this being combined with family commitments, involvement in sport was a reason for non-attendance. The authors comment that, for women, barriers to attendance tend to act in concert, with husbands being unable to provide transport and baby-sit at the same time. Childcare provision was found to be the most important factor that would make attendance easier, particularly for single parents. Thus, the evidence suggests that, although women would value the opportunities that distance learning provides, lack of support for learning is often a factor that may be detrimental to their progress. If support could be provided, distance learning could offer women an important opportunity for further and higher education, and this will be subject of the concluding section of this chapter.

Distance learning opportunities for women

In concluding this chapter, it is useful to consider the availability of distance learning opportunities and the different purposes they might serve. Many institutions of further and higher education provide a range of distance learning modules as part of their portfolio of courses. Most of these will cover the different academic levels from sub-degree level, certificate level (level I), diploma level (level II), degree level (level III) to Master's degree (level IV). The different levels are likely to be used for different purposes. As the research for this book was based on diploma level modules, these will be the focus of this chapter.

Diploma level distance learning modules often consist of a series of modules from which students can select, in order to build up sufficient academic credit to access a degree course. When used for this purpose only, students are normally not restricted in selecting their modules, except by the obvious restriction of the number of modules available. An additional restriction may be imposed, however, if a particular module is required in order to access a specified degree programme. In situations where students are collecting credits to access a degree programme, a diploma is often not awarded, since a specified award would require a particular portfolio of modules. There are variations, however, within different institutions, with some offering a Diploma in Higher Education to students who can demonstrate that they have successfully completed the requisite number of modules at the required level.

Degree level and Master's degree level distance learning modules tend not to be used for 'access' purposes and, normally, form part of a coherent award. There are, generally, three variations in the use of distance learning within degree and Master's degree awards, reflecting the three common modes of study:

- class-based study—in class-based study, distance learning materials may be used as part of the teaching resource
- mixed mode—mixed mode programmes of study involve a mixture of modules, some being taught by class-based teaching, and others being distance learning modules
- distance learning—some institutions offer degrees or Master's degrees that are studied purely by distance learning.

Selecting the appropriate mode of study for personal learning needs and circumstances is a crucial part of the learning process. Students often select distance learning courses because they are the only ones available, or because they are unable to attend the institution on specified days. These are very sound reasons, but it is important to find out what support is offered by the institution, whether attendance at the institution is required, and whether the course relies on paper-based learning materials, or whether it is delivered on-line, thereby requiring access to a computer and computer familiarity. There are numerous factors to consider before embarking on a distance learning course. These will be discussed throughout this book; for example, there is a need to consider, whether:

- distance learning matches your own learning characteristics
- you are likely to adopt an appropriate approach to study to be a successful distance learner
- you can access the appropriate type and level of support
- you are able to use the resources at your disposal to develop coping strategies that enable you to be successful.

Summary

This chapter has considered the value of distance learning and the opportunities it can provide. The nature of distance learning reveals important characteristics, which highlight important distinctions between distance learning and class-based learning. The concept of student independence is of particular importance to distance learning, particularly in relation to how this is fostered by the role of the tutor and the individual needs of students. The needs of women as distance learners are of particular significance, since distance learning is a popular mode of study for women learners. The chapter concludes with examples of the opportunities that distance learning might offer women who wish to use this mode of study.

Reflection

This section is designed to provide the opportunity for personal reflection on the content of the chapter and how it can be applied to your personal plans for further study. A series of questions are provided to facilitate this process.

- In considering the advantages and limitations of distance learning (see *Table 1.1*), does it appear to have sufficient benefit for you as a means of pursuing further study?
- Consider again the differences between distance learning and class-based study. Which of the characteristics of each mode of study identified in *Table 1.2* appeal to you?
- How prepared do you feel to challenge the conventional (passive) role of student, in favour of negotiating an independent role with the help of a tutor?
- If you are female, how closely does your situation mirror that described in this chapter?

Practical activity

If you think that distance learning might have some benefit in helping you to engage in further study, contact your nearest further or higher education institution and find out what distance learning provision they can offer.

References

Bailey D (1992) Facilitator not teacher: A role for tutors in open learning nurse education. *J Adv Nurs* **17**: 983–91

Burge L (1988) Beyond androgogy: Some explorations for distance learning design. *J Dist Educ* **3**(1): 5–23

Chene A (1983) The concept of autonomy in adult education: A philosophical discussion. Adult Educ Q 34(1): 47–83

Chesterton P (1985) Curriculum control in distance education. *Teach Dist* **26**: 32–7

Cropley AJ, Kahl TN (1983) Distance education and distance learning: some psychological considerations. *Dist Educ* **4**(1):27–39

Cunningham I (1987) Openness and learning to learn. In: Hodgson V, Mann S, Snell B (eds). *Beyond Distance Teaching Towards Open Learning*. Open University Press, Buckingham: 40–59

Diaz DP, Cartnal RB (1999) Students' learning styles in two classes: Online distance learning and equivalent on-campus. *Coll Teach* **47**(4): 130–5

Evans T, Nation D (1989) Dialogue in practice, research and theory in distance education. *Open Learn* **4**(2): 37–42

Gibbs G, Lockwood F, Morgan A, Taylor E (1982) Student learning and course design 1: In-text devices in Open University texts. *Study Methods Group Report*, No. 12. Institute of Educational Technology, Open University, Milton Keynes

Green CP (1987) Multiple role women: The real world of the mature RN learner. *J Nurs Educ* **26**(7): 266–71

Harris D (1976) Educational technology at the Open University: A short history of achievement and cancellation. *Br J Educat Tech* **71**: 44

Holmberg B (1989) *Theory and Practice of Distance Education.* Routledge, London

Keegan D (1985) On defining distance education. In: Sewart D, Keegan D, Holmberg B (eds). *Distance Education: International Perspectives.* Croom Helm, Beckenham, Kent

Keegan DJ (1980) On defining distance education. *Dist Educ* **1**(1): 13–36

Kirkup G, von Prummer C (1990) Support and connectedness: The needs of women distance education students. *J Dist Educ* **5**(2): 9–31

Leornard A, Jowett J (1990) *Project 2000—1, Charting the Course: A Study of 6 ENB Pilot Schemes in Pre-registration Nurse Education.* National Foundation for Educational Research in England and Wales, Slough

Naylor P, Cowie H, Stevenson K (1990) Using student and tutor perspectives in the development of open tutoring. *Open Learn* **5**(1): 9–18

Perraton H (1983) A theory of distance education. In: Sewart D, Keegan D, Holmberg B (eds). *Distance Education: International Perspectives.* Croom Helm, Beckenham, Kent: 34–45

Pym FR, Atkinson AM (1990) Reaching out via distance education to nurses: Needs assessment, planning and implications. Paper presented at the third congress of the Canadian Association for Distance Education, Quebec City. In: Pym FR (1992) Women and distance education: a nursing perspective. *J Adv Nurs* **17**: 383–9

Pym FR (1992) Women and distance education: a nursing perspective. *J Adv Nurs* **17**: 383–9

Rogers WS (1986) Changing attitudes through distance learning, *Open Learn* **1**(3): 12–17

Rumble G (1989) Open learning, distance learning, and the misuse of language'. *Open Learn* **4** (2): 28–36

Sewart D (1987) Limitations of the Learning Package. In: Thorpe M, Grugeon D, (eds). *Open Learning for Adults,* Longman, Harlow: 31–7

Snell RS, Hodgson VE, Mann SJ (1987) Beyond distance teaching towards open learning. In: Hodgson V, Mann S, Snell B (eds). *Beyond Distance Teaching Towards Open Learning.* Open University Press, Milton Keynes: 161–72

Stewart A (1985) Appropriate educational technology: Does "appropriateness" have implications for the theoretical framework of educational technology? *Educat Comm Tech J* **33**: 58–65

Tait A (1988) Democracy in distance education and the role of tutorial and counselling services. *J Dist Educ* **3**(1): 95–9

United Kingdom Central Council for Nursing, Midwifery and Health Visiting (1994) *The Future of Professional Practice: The Council's Standards for Education and Practice Following Registration.* UKCC, London

Von Prummer C, Rossie U (1988) Gender in distance education at the Fern Universitat. *Open Learn* **3**(2): 3–12

Wedemeyer CA (1977) Independent study. In: Knowles A.S, (ed). *The International Encyclopaedia of Higher Education*. CIHED, Boston

2
Student characteristics: learning styles, strategies, approaches and preferences

Introduction

The research on which this book is based revealed that distance learning students use different strategies when studying materials. These strategies depend to a large extent on individual characteristics, such as learning style, approaches to study and learning preferences. There is a vast amount of literature concerning learning styles, strategies, approaches to study and learning preferences, and these will be explored in this chapter. Understanding such theories enables curriculum developers to address issues, such as how individual learning styles can be used to improve the learning experience, how deep learning can be ensured, and identifying the barriers to learning (Lockitt, 1999). This chapter reviews the literature relating to individual student characteristics and considers its application to distance learning. The chapter begins with definitions of terms relating to individual characteristics. It is then divided into sections covering learning style theory, as well as theories around approaches to study and learning preferences. The chapter concludes with a reflective activity and a practical activity.

Definitions of terms

Success in distance learning depends, in part, on the different ways in which students learn. These differences include the following:

- learning styles
- learning strategies
- approaches to study

- study preferences.

Brief definitions of these characteristics are presented in *Table 2.1.*

Table 2.1: Different learning characteristics and their definitions

Learning characteristics	Definition
Learning styles	A habitual preference for using particular abilities to make sense of information, including problem solving, thinking, perceiving, and remembering
Learning strategies	Ways of approaching learning that vary with the task and may be learned and developed
Approaches to study	Includes a variety of learning styles and strategies that can be modified by external constraints, including those arising from the institution, as well as the student. These factors impact on students' motivation to study, which, in turn, influences their approach to learning and learning strategy
Study preferences	The propensity of an individual to choose a particular instructional techniques

Learning style has been defined as a habitual preference for using particular abilities and processing information. Some authors, such as Sternberg (1990), argue that learning styles will vary across tasks and situations, whereas others, such as Riding (1997) and Tennant (1988), believe that learning style is relatively fixed.

Riding and Rayner (1998:11) offer distinctions between 'learning styles' and 'learning strategies' as follows:

> *'... style probably has a physiological basis and is fairly fixed for the individual. By contrast, strategies are ways that may be learned and developed to cope with situations and tasks, and particularly methods of utilising styles to make the best of situations for which the styles are not ideally suited.'*

Learning strategies are seen, then, as deliberate methods employed by people to compensate for the limitations of their usual learning style. Strategies are not always needed, however, since an individual's normal style might be quite appropriate for a particular task. Sternberg (1990) develops this view, suggesting that styles are not better or worse, but rather matters of fit, i.e. fitting the style to the particular task and situation. According to Sternberg (1990), some tasks require detailed orientation and others require global holistic orientation. Furthermore, people differ in their strengths and flexibility of stylistic preferences, some being particularly strong and relatively inflexible, others being more adaptable. Styles are socialised and so can change across the life span with changing demands of life (Sternberg, 1990). Readers may wish to consider their own style and strategy in past learning situations (see *Box 2.1a and b*).

Box 2.1a: Your learning style

- Consider your last learning situation
- Can you recall how you went about learning?
- Did you focus in on fine details or did you take in a broad picture, scanning text and ignoring the finer details?
- Does this differ from the way in which you approach learning now?
- Do you generally change your learning style to meet the demands of different situations, or does it remain the same?
- If you think back over the past 10 years, do you think your learning *style* has changed, or remained static?

Box 2.1b: Your learning strategy

- Consider some of the learning strategies you have used in the past
- Have you developed different strategies during periods of study to enable you to learn more effectively?
- Do you, for example, take short cuts when reading to ensure you read only what is relevant?
- Have the strategies you used differed according to the learning task?
- Have your learning strategies been successful?
- Do you think there is a 'fit' between the nature of the task and the learning strategy adopted?

Research into learning styles

Research into learning styles has its roots in psychology and centres on cognition, personality and activity (Grigerenko and Sternberg, 1995). Attempts have been made to clarify the confusing terminology, by classifying the various theories (Curry, 1983; Sadler-Smith, 1997). Curry used the analogy of an onion in which the various layers reflect three groupings of cognitive/learning styles (see *Figure 2.1*). The outer layer refers to *instructional preference,* such as choice of learning environment, e.g., a classroom, or a quiet room in a library. This layer is most visible, as it is closest to the outside world. The middle layer, *information processing,* refers to the way in which individuals assimilate information. This layer does not involve the environment as it is concerned with what goes on in people's heads. It is, however, modifiable by learning strategies, such as deliberate attempts to focus in on detail, rather than attempting to take in the whole picture. The innermost layer, *cognitive personality type,* refers to the adaptation and assimilation of information. This layer is considered to be permanent and apparent only when behaviour is observed across many learning instances. It is, therefore, not subject to changes resulting from the adoption of different strategies.

An alternative to Curry's classification is Sadler-Smith's (1996) four broad categories of learning (learning preferences, learning styles, approaches to studying, and cognitive styles). These have similarity with, but extend, Curry's classification. Most of the literature on learning styles and strategies can be located somewhere within Curry's model and Sadler-Smith's four categories.

In view of the lack of a conclusive categorisation system, this chapter will adapt Curry's Onion Model, using Sadler-Smith's approaches to study as an additional layer. Learning preferences will be used rather than instructional preferences, as this seems more consistent with a distance learning philosophy. External factors, outside the layers of the onion, are also additional to Curry's model. Thus, the framework that will underpin this chapter is presented in *Figure 2.1*.

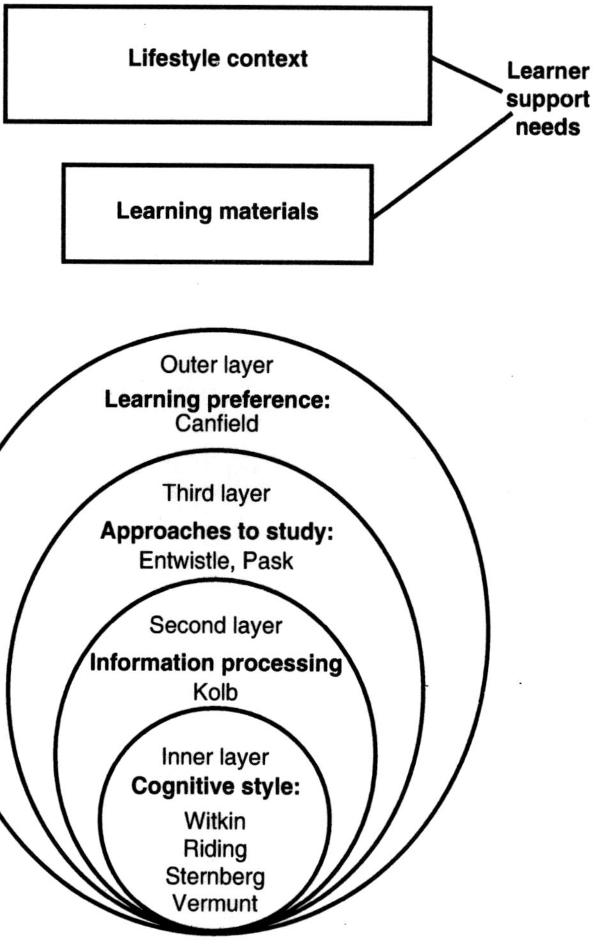

Figure 2.1: An adaptation of Curry's Onion Model (reproduced with kind permission from Curry L (1983) *An Organisation of Learning Styles and Theory Constructs*. ERIC Document, 235, 185)

The different layers of styles and strategies are seen as being impacted on by the demands of both the learning materials and student lifestyle commitments. Learning support needs to act as a mediating factor between the outside world and learning styles and strategies in that, given the appropriate support, students can compensate for lack of compatibility between their own learning style and strategies and how these interact with the learning materials and personal lifestyle factors. This has particular relevance to distance learning, due to the complex relationship that exists between learning styles and approaches to learning within a wider societal context of adult learners.

The following section explains *Figure 2.1*, beginning with the inner layer of the onion (cognitive style), moving on to the second layer (information processing), then to the third layer (approaches to study), and, finally, to the outer layer (learning preferences).

Cognitive style

There are a number of style characteristics that can be included within the cognitive style theory. These are:

- serialist/analytic versus holist/global dimensions (Pask and Scott, 1972)
- perceptual functioning (Witkin *et al*, 1977)
- impulsivity-reflectivity (Kagan *et al*, 1964)
- thinking styles (Sternberg, 1990)
- style-directedness (Vermunt, 1996).

Each of these will be dealt with separately.

Serialist/analytic-holist/global dimensions

Serialist and analytic learners are not dissimilar to each other. In describing the serialist learner, Pask and Scott (1972) outline how such students learn, remember, and recapitulate by relating items of information in the form of simple data links. In addition, they tend to assimilate lengthy sequences of data and are, therefore, intolerant of irrelevant information.

This can be compared with people who have an extreme analytic style, who:

> *'. . . have focussed attention, noticing and remembering details. They have an interest in operations and procedures and proper ways of doing things, and prefer step-by-step sequential learning.... They are gifted at critical, logical thinking' (Schmeck, 1988: 328).*

Analytics will be self-reliant, consistent, idealistic, and organised (Riding, 1991), and information does not need to be either concrete or connected to their personal experience (Flannery, 1993). If left to their own devices, analytic learners will make sense of information by sequentially focussing in on details and unpacking them. By comparison, serialists attempt to build understanding, focussing on details and logical relationships between argument and evidence, and on operations taken strictly in a linear sequence (Pask and Scott, 1972). It is clear, therefore, that there are fewer differences than similarities between analytic and serialist learners. Indeed, sequential serialist learning could be a deliberate *strategy* adopted by analytic learners to enable them to approach the task logically.

Analytic and serialist learners differ fundamentally from holist learners in that holists process information as a whole, whereas analytics process information in parts, so that it can be broken down and analysed. Holist (global) learners start with the whole picture, so that they can get the gist of things. They make sense of information by scanning, to form overall impressions. They process information simultaneously, ideas and experiences being seen all at once, rather than in any particular order (Flannery, 1993). According to Le Cornu (1999), global learners have been labelled as 'passive' or 'spectator' learners since they allow relevant features of a topic to emerge of their own accord, rather than working with material in order to determine the features themselves.

Unlike analytic learners, who do not require learning to be related to their personal experience, learners who process information globally (holists) need information to be connected to their personal experiences or they will discard it as unimportant (Flannery, 1993). Their thinking is more intuitive and they are more impulsive than analytic learners (Schmeck, 1988).

Each of these two opposing learning styles has its own advantages and disadvantages (Cooper, 1977). Holists have an unclear concept of boundaries, poor sequential learning and memory, poor organisation and reading/writing skills, and poor timekeeping. They are inconsistent with progress, difficult to monitor and are often late bloomers (Cooper, 1977). Since schools often emphasise an analytical approach (Flannery, 1993), adult learners who find themselves in settings that perpetuate a school structure may find learning difficult.

Holists might, however, draw on the strengths of their learning style, such as creativity, improvisation, lateral thinking and problem solving, so that they can understand the whole task rather than merely isolated elements of it (Cooper, 1977).

Cooper also suggests that there could be conflict between the way in which students think and the way in which they process information. Students who think in terms of visual images, for example, might be disadvantaged by the need to process information sequentially when studying distance learning packages. This is because sequential learning might cause them to lose some of the advantages of their learning style (e.g. creativity, flexibility, making unusual connections) and to acquire some of the disadvantages of the sequential serialist style (e.g. regurgitation, difficulty making decisions without clear evidence, inability to transfer skills). The design of distance learning materials is, therefore, important if it is to meet the needs of different students. For this reason, many distance learning texts include information presented visually as well as in text form.

Perceptual functioning

In studies investigating how students perceive in learning situations, Witkin *et al* (1977) identify distinctions between field dependent and field independent students. Their study used an 'embedded-figures test' to determine the extent to which the 'surrounding organised field has influenced the person's perception of an item within it' (Witkin *et al*, 1977: 6). Each subject was scored according to the time taken to locate a simple figure within the complex design. The ability to locate this figure quickly was considered to be comparable to thinking analytically. Witkin *et al* described subjects whose perception was dominated by the background as field dependent, since the prevailing 'field' dominated their perception. By comparison, subjects who perceived items as separate from the background were labelled as field independent. The authors cited a number of studies that identify further characteristics of field dependent and field independent people. For example, field dependent people attend to social cues that include facial expression and verbal messages with social content, and are described as having a 'with-people' orientation (Witkin *et al*, 1977). By comparison, field independent people 'are more likely to be aware of needs, feelings, attributes, which they experience as their own and as distinct from those of others' (Witkin *et al*, 1977: 13). They prefer to work in a solitary manner and appreciate abstract content.

It is likely that distance learning will demand some of the characteristics of field independence, as defined by Witkin *et al* (1977). Such characteristics include:

- ability to work in a solitary manner
- self-definition of goals
- intrinsic reinforcement
- a preference for students to structure their own work.

Indeed, independent learners are, arguably, more suited to distance education (James and Gardner, 1995), and have been more successful in telecourses than dependent learners (Gee, 1990). Moreover, in a recent comparison between online and campus students, distance students more strongly favoured independent learning styles (Diaz and Cartnal, 1999). By comparison, field dependent students prefer group work, to interact more frequently with peers and teachers, and require extrinsic reinforcement and direction (Witkin *et al*, 1977), situations that are limited in distance education.

Impulsivity-reflexivity

The impulsivity-reflectivity dimension of cognitive style (Kagan *et al*, 1964) refers to students who are impulsive in the way in which they study, and those who are reflective. Cognitively impulsive students reach decisions quickly after a brief review of opinions, whereas cognitively reflective students deliberate before making a response. The instrument to measure this style—the Matching Familiar Figures Test—has been used by a series of investigators and has demonstrated stability over time and with different tasks (Riding and Rayner, 1998). However, Jones (1997) argues that the impulsivity-reflectivity dimension is more susceptible to change by internal and external influences, such as constraints of time or competing commitments. For this reason, Jones argues, impulsivity-reflectivity may be more appropriately defined as a strategy, rather than a learning style, since it is open to the influence of factors, such as motivation and emotion. In distance education settings, cognitively impulsive learners might be expected to adopt a different approach to the learning materials than students who are cognitively reflective. Indeed, emotion and motivation could be significant factors to women distance learners placed in a position of using distance learning to advance their careers. Decisions to either use materials reflectively or impulsively could, therefore, be part of a learning strategy.

Cognitive styles are summarised in the following reflective activity, following which thinking styles will be discussed.

Reflective activity

Before moving on the look at thinking styles in the next section, review the characteristics of the cognitive styles discussed above (see *Table 2.2*). Consider which of the styles matches your own style of learning most closely. It might be that more than one style characterises your own style of learning. How compatible is your style with distance learning? What challenges are you likely to face if you follow a distance learning programme of study?

Table 2.2: Characteristics of different cognitive styles

Serialist/analytic	Holist
Links information together in lengthy sequences	Processes information as a whole
Intolerant of irrelevant information	No order to processing of information
Focussed—remembers details	Needs concrete examples to relate to personal experience
Follows procedures	
Step-by-step	Scans materials to form overall impressions
Logical	Intuitive and impulsive
Organised	Unclear concept of boundaries
No requirement for concrete examples	Poor sequential learning and memory, poor organisation and reading/writing skills, and poor timekeeping

Serialist/analytic	Holist
Tends to regurgitate	Inconsistent with progress and difficult to monitor
Finds difficulty making decisions without clear evidence	Creative
Unable to transfer skills	Able to improvise
Good at problem solving	Thinks laterally
Field dependence	**Field independence**
When faced with ambiguity, adheres to what is presented	When faced with ambiguity, restructures material presented
Prefers working in groups and to interact with peers and teachers,	Able to define own goals
Requires extrinsic reinforcement and direction	Relies on intrinsic reinforcement
Attends to social cues (facial/verbal expression)	Prefers to structure own work
With-people orientation	Perceives own needs/feelings as distinct from others
	Likes solitary activity and abstract content
Impulsive	**Reflective**
Reviews opinions and reaches decisions quickly	Deliberates before responding
Open to influence of motivation and emotion	Open to influence of motivation and emotion

Thinking styles

Sternberg (1990) identified a theory of mental self-government based on the premise that people need to manage their everyday activities. Since there are many ways of doing this, people try to adapt themselves to the stylistic demands of a given situation, by choosing styles of managing themselves with which they feel comfortable. The significance of this theory to distance education is that students are likely to adapt their style of self-management to the particular demands of the distance learning situation. Sternberg went on to identify *functions, scope, forms and levels* of self-government.

Functions of self-government

Sternberg (1990) identified three functions, which mirror the government of people:

- legislative (concerned with creating, formulating, imagining and planning)
- executive (concerned with implementing and doing)
- judicial (concerned with judging, evaluating, and comparing).

Although people use all three of these functions, they will have a proclivity for one. People with a proclivity for the *legislative function* like to create their own rules or structures, like doing things their own way, and welcome problems and materials that lack structure and demand creativity. The flexible nature of distance education could, therefore, provide an opportunity for such students to impose their own structure on the learning task. By comparison, people in whom the *executive function* dominates like to follow guidelines, to be told what to do, and for problems to be well-structured and spelled out for them. Such students would probably need a high level of structure imposed in distance learning situations, both in terms of materials and institutional support mechanisms. The *judicial function* is characterised by a preference to evaluate facts and procedures and to write critiques, rather than coming up with their own ideas. Such students in distance learning would probably prefer well-structured packages, but would follow guidelines and procedures, and provide critiques with minimal institutional support.

Scope of self-government

Sternberg's (1990) *scope* of mental self-government is divided into internal and external. Internal self-government involves tasks in which students work on their own, such as distance learning. External self-government involves working with other people. This could create conflict for distance learners with this type of mental self-government, as opportunities to work with others are limited.

Forms of self-government

The *forms of self-government* comprise *monarchic, hierarchic, oligarchic,* and *anarchic*. In the *monarchic* form of self-government, a single goal predominates, and the student pursues, single-mindedly, one goal at a time. By comparison, the *hierarchic* form is characterised by pursuit of multiple goals, which students prioritise in order to focus in on the specific and relevant information. This would, possibly, enable the woman distance learner to prioritise the multiple tasks of domestic and work life in a manner that also allows her time to study. Students favouring the *oligarchic* form also pursue multiple goals, but have difficulty in prioritising and, therefore, experience conflict that prevents them completing tasks because they cannot decide which is the most important. *Anarchic* students take a random approach, are intolerant of rules and regulations, and resist authority.

Most education institutions reward the executive/hierarchic style (Sternberg, 1990). Distance learning, however, requires the use of judicial and legislative functions as well as executive. Judicial functions would involve evaluating theories presented in learning materials, and making judgements about what is relevant to an assignment. Legislative functions would involve working creatively and using the flexibility provided by distance learning to create their own rules. The forms of mental self-government required by distance learning tend towards *oligarchic,* in that students probably prioritise between reading materials, gathering information towards the assignment, and writing the assignment. Each of these elements takes priority at different times, but also competes with other demands from work and domestic life.

Levels of self-government

The *level of self-governance* (Sternberg, 1990) resembles serialist/holist learning (Pask and Scott, 1972) in that it refers to global and local processing. Global processing problems require abstract (holistic) thinking. Local processing requires concrete thinking in which detail is appreciated. Sternberg suggests that people become more global with age and experience. Thus, adult distance learners might be more holistic in information processing.

According to Sternberg (1996), lectures cater for the executive/hierarchical needs of students. Small group discussions respond to external/judicial styles, while required reading caters for a slightly wider range of needs. Reading for detail, in particular, would appeal to local/executive styles, while reading for main ideas would cater for global/executive styles, and reading for analysis (the desired outcome) would respond to judicial styles. Indeed, different elements of assignments require different forms of self-government, as indicated in *Table 2.3*.

Table 2.3: Self-governance required for different assignment tasks

Requirement of assignment	Self-governance required	Example
Analysis	Judicial *function*	Evaluating theories and deciding what to include in assignment
Creativity	Legislative *function*	Planning assignment and formulating arguments
Organisation	Hierarchical *form*	Prioritising reading against note taking, writing assignment
Time allocation	Hierarchical *form*	Prioritising assignment work against work and domestic commitments
Working alone	Internal *scope*	Working independently without discussion with others

As can be seen in *Table 2.2*, the type of assignments used in distance learning demand a high degree of adaptation across the different functions, forms and scope of self-government (Sternberg, 1996). Sternberg (1988) comments that gender and occupation may also influence style. He proposes that the legislative style has been more acceptable in men than women, men setting the rules and women following. This might be prevalent, then, in female occupations, such as health care, in which the dominant profession (medicine) is likely to be controlled by males. This might perpetuate the executive style and inhibit adaptation to alternatives.

Style-directedness

Vermunt (1994; 1998) developed an Inventory of Learning Styles (ILS) in which he identified four styles of learning as follows:

- undirected
- reproduction-directed
- meaning-directed
- application-directed.

This approach to the analysis of style is particularly valuable, due to its intention to cross the barriers between cognitive styles, strategies, approaches to learning and learning preferences.

The *undirected* learning style has similarities with the *oligarchic form* of self-government (Sternberg, 1990). It is characterised by difficulty in selecting the most important parts in study materials and distinguishing between major and minor points. Everything being of equal importance, such students do not know what they have to remember, while study materials often are too voluminous to remember everything (Vermunt, 1996). Such students are unable to apply learning to real life. They regulate their learning by following instructional directions, but have a precarious hold on them. This approach, according Vermetten *et al* (1999), is similar to Tait and Entwistle's (1996) apathetic approach.

Undirected learners focus strongly on the assignment, and adjust to difficult concepts by reading and re-reading. They realise, however, that their current learning styles do not suffice, but do not know how to approach their studies in a better way, and become concerned that they cannot learn the study materials. Consequently, they lack confidence and worry about their achievements. Mental modes of learning associated with undirected learners comprise a preference for external regulation (such as assignment guidance) and the belief that teachers and course writers should sum up what students need to know, show clear relations between concepts, and sketch an overview of contents.

The undirected style has clear implications for distance learning. According to Vermunt (1996), undirected learners need teachers to explain how they should study, and explicate difficult parts of assignments until students understand them. Co-operation with other students was also seen as important, to give them support and help with motivation. This would indicate the need for self-help groups and group tutorials for undirected learners in distance education.

The *meaning-directed* style differs considerably from the undirected style, in that such students extract content from learning materials, if they have an intrinsic interest for them. In doing so, they ignore fine details, and focus on the 'meaning' of the content, which is often reflected in central themes and concepts. Once they have identified the central concepts, they interrelate them to try to build up a complete picture and often approach material critically, by asking questions about it so that they can form their own impressions. As well as actively selecting from, and restructuring materials, these students consult non-prescribed literature in order to deepen their interest. If they encounter difficulty in learning, they find out for themselves where the problem occurred, and analyse the situation in order to solve it. In some respects, meaning directed learners have some similarity with Sternberg's (1990; 1996) legislative *function* (creating their own rules) and internal *scope* (working alone) of self-government. In addition to its similarity with Sternberg's legislative function, the meaning-directed style has also been described as similar to Entwistle's (1988) meaning orientation (Vermetten *et al*, 1999).

The *reproduction-directed* learning style is characterised by selecting and underlining the main parts of the materials (Vermunt, 1996), and resembles Entwistle's (1988) reproducing orientation (Vermetten *et al*, 1999). Students with this learning style follow the advice of course writers in distinguishing major and minor points and have little difficulty making selections. They appear to adopt a serialist approach to learning (Pask, 1976) by learning sequentially, step-by-step, part by part, studying every topic separately. They also resemble the executive function of self-government (Sternberg, 1990) by consulting no other sources than the course materials and following instructions. Reproductive learners seldom reflect on their learning or find out for themselves the cause of their difficulties. As Vermunt (1996) points out, these students tend to be insecure and underline text excessively because they feel they need to know everything. They like structured, small segments in materials and do not wish to discuss things with other students. For these students, the teacher is there to clarify points, and generate interest as necessary.

The cognitive processing involved in the *application-diected* learning style is concerned with usefulness of learning content and realising personal goals (Vermunt, 1996). Such students have similarities with Sternberg's (1990) judicial function of self-government, in that they select their reading according to its practical relevance, and search for relations between the subject matter and the reality to which it refers. Application-directed learners regulate their learning by consulting other books when they experience difficulty, make schemes and resort to an analytic strategy. They do nothing with materials that do not interest them, viewing knowledge as present only if it can be used. These students are vocationally orientated, and want to learn a profession and acquire professional skills.

Before considering some of the studies using Vermunt's styles, readers may wish to engage in a reflective activity to review the styles in relation to their own learning.

Reflective activity

The main characteristics described by Vermunt (1996) are listed in *Table 2.4*. Consider which of Vermunt's styles of learning most closely matches your own. How compatible is your style with distance learning? What challenges is it likely to present?

Table 2.4: Descriptions of Vermunt's (1996) four styles of learning

Undirected	Meaning-directed
Difficulty in selection of reading	Extract what is of personal interest from materials
Unable to apply reading to real life	Ignore fine details and focus on central themes and concepts
Follow directions but find this difficult	Interrelate concepts to build picture
Focus on assignment	Read critically by asking questions to form own interpretation
Read and re-read to facilitate understanding	Actively select from, and structure materials
Concerned about ability to cope with, and understand materials	Consult additional reading
Lack confidence and worry about achievements	Diagnose and solve own learning problems
Need assignment guidance	
Need help in making links between concepts	
Reproduction-directed	**Application-directed**
Select main points by underlining	Select reading for its practical relevance
Follow advice of course writers	Search for relations between subject matter and reality
Learn sequentially, step-by-step	
Do not consult additional materials	Consult other books when in difficulty and make schemes and analyse
Do not reflect on learning or diagnose causes of problems	Do nothing with materials that do not interest them
Feel they need to know everything	View knowledge as existing only if it can be used
Like structure and clear segments in materials	Vocationally orientated
Do not wish to discuss with other students	
Teacher role is clarificatory	

It is generally thought that, of the four styles identified by Vermunt, the meaning-directed and application-directed are the most desirable and that these styles will increase with experience. Three similar studies have been conducted to test these assumptions using Vermunt's ILS (Busato *et al*, 1998; Vermetten *et al*, 1999). Busato *et al* conducted two studies, a cross-sectional study of 800 students from years one to five and a longitudinal study that followed a cohort of students. Vermetten *et al* conducted a longitudinal study (involving 861 freshmen and 524 second year students) using the ILS on students from law, economics, social sciences, language and literature. Although the response rates for the studies were low (approximately 20%, for Busato *et al*'s studies and 42% and 31% respectively for Vermetten *et al*'s), there was some agreement between them. Busato *et al*'s cross-sectional study failed to confirm their hypothesis that application- and meaning-directed styles would increase in later years, and that undirected and reproduction learning styles would decrease. This finding was contradicted, however, by both Busato *et al*'s and Vermetten *et al*'s longitudinal studies, which reported an increase in use of the meaning-directed style as students progressed through their study. Busato *et al* also reported an increase in application-directed scores over the years, while the undirected and reproduction-directed scores decreased. This latter finding is at odds with Vermetten *et al*'s study, which found that reproduction-directed styles did not decrease during the programme of study. The evidence is unclear,therefore, regarding the effect of progression through study on students' style-directedness, although there seems to be a trend towards students attending to the *meaning* of subject matter and applying themselves more to study as they gain in experience.

These are interesting findings, particularly when considered in the light of the impact style-directedness might have on academic success. Busato *et al* tested Vermunt's style theory for its relationship to academic success and found a negative correlation between undirected style and academic success in second, third, and fourth year students. This suggests that students using an undirected style would be less successful academically.

The discussion of the inner layer of Curry's Onion Model, which includes cognitive styles, thinking styles, and style-directedness, is now complete. The next section will move to the second layer of the onion.

Information processing

Information processing represents the second layer of the onion in *Figure 2.1.* It overlaps with cognitive style since reference is made to the way in which students' thinking influences the manner in which they process information (Cooper, 1977). Thinking, however, being concerned with cognition, is suitably placed in the inner layer of the onion.

Kolb (1976) defines learning style as a preferred way of processing information from the world. People may process information in either an *abstract* or a *concrete* manner (see *Figure 2.2*). *Abstract* processing involves thinking about and analysing abstract theories. Students who process information in this way do not need practical examples and are satisfied with a theoretical text. By comparison, students who process information in a *concrete* manner benefit from texts that include practical examples, such as case studies. By working with concrete examples, such students are able to link abstract theory to their own personal experience and this process facilitates their understanding.

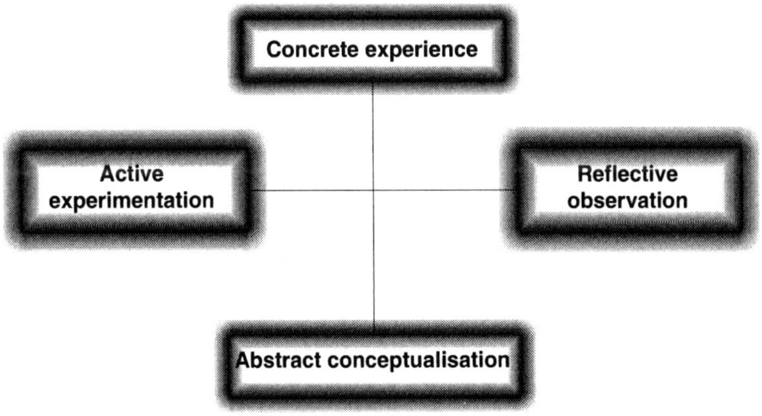

Figure 2.2: Kolb's two dimensions (Kolb 1976)

The *reflection observation* versus active *experiment dimension* of Kolb's model (*Figure* 2.2) refers to how individuals *transform* the experiences they have in order to make sense of them. Reflective thinkers are said to transform experience *internally* by reflection, whereas active thinkers transform experience *externally*, by actively manipulating the environment. Kolb designed a Learning Style Inventory (LSI) to measure these information-processing styles in students.

Kolb's LSI comprises a four stage cycle, building on the two dimensions in *Figure* 2.2. Within the cycle (*Figure* 2.3) individuals begin by using their concrete experience to reflect on. This reflection on concrete observations (reflective observation) enables them to understand the *meaning* of the learning experience, which they use to form abstract concepts (abstract conceptualisation). Individuals then use these abstract conceptualisations to generate theories and hypotheses. Once theories and hypotheses are formulated, individuals use active experimentation to test them in new situations. This whole process results in the solving of problems.

As can be seen in *Figure* 2.2 and *Figure* 2.3, two polar opposites are evident in the cycle. Concrete experience is the polar opposite of abstract conceptualisation and reflective observation is the opposite of active experimentation. From these dimensions Kolb (1976) identified four statistically significant learning styles as follows:

- convergers
- divergers
- assimilators
- accommodators.

Again, the learning styles are polar opposites, divergers being opposite to convergers and assimilators opposite to accommodators (see *Figure* 2.3).

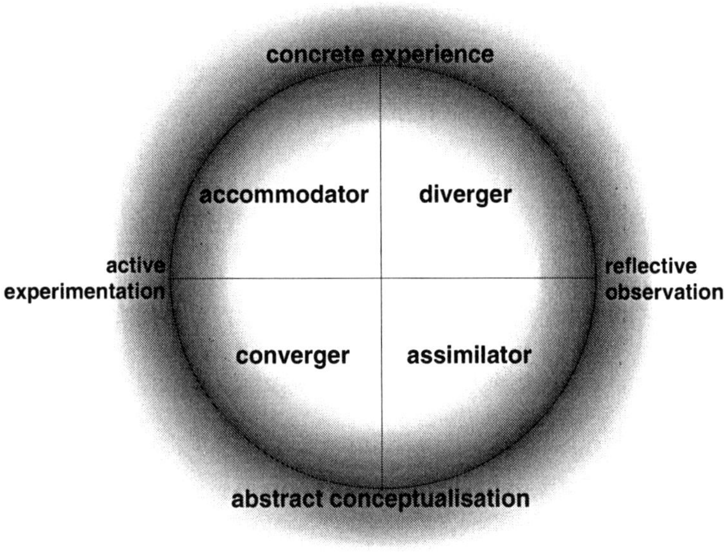

Figure 2.3: Kolb's learning styles (Kolb 1976)

Divergers favour both concrete experience and reflective observation. They are imaginative and view situations from multiple perspectives. They prefer concrete, people-orientated learning experiences in which they can 'brain storm' new ideas. In distance learning situations, they may be expected to prefer concrete examples in the text and face-face tutorials in which they can brain storm ideas (Carnwell, 1996).

Assimilators prefer reflective observation and abstract conceptualisation. They are orientated towards theoretical models, inductive reasoning and learning experiences requiring symbolic thought. Their lack of interest in people may make them natural distance learners, since they require little more than text materials to reflect upon and analyse (Carnwell, 1996).

Convergers prefer abstract conceptualisation and active experimentation. They are good at testing out theories in practical situations and problem solving, and prefer learning situations requiring the search for a single correct answer. They tend to be unemotional, uninterested in people and have narrow technical interests. As distance learners, convergers can be expected to focus only on parts of the text that can be applied to practice and provide specific answers. During group tutorials, they will require a single solution to problems rather than discussion of theories or group support. They may be instrumental and assessment-orientated in their learning, and may restrict their reading of distance learning materials to information that will enable them to complete an assignment (Carnwell, 1996).

Accommodators prefer concrete experience and active experimentation, and excel at carrying out plans and seeking new experiences. They are less analytical than others and trust their instinct in problem solving situations. They solve problems in an intuitive trial-and-error manner, relying heavily on other people rather than on their own analytic ability. They are generally well-organised and systematic in distance learning situations, although their competence in using concrete experience and their lack of analytical skills may result in a need for tutorial support (Carnwell, 1996).

Probably due to the popularity of Kolb's LSI, a number of studies have been conducted to test its validity. Hunsaker (1981) reviewed seven of these studies and found that two studies (Kolb, 1973; Carlson *et al*, 1979) showed the LSI to have high predictive validity; two (Kevin *et al*, 1975; Plovnick, 1975) reported validity on one dimension and the other three (Reifle and Edwards, 1975; Wunderlick and Gjierdi, 1978; Freedman and Stumpf, 1978) concluded that it had no predictive validity. Although Hunsaker concludes that the LSI is invalid, he does acknowledge that there is considerable support for the learning model itself. Riding and Rayner (1998), who question whether the model is a description of a specific cycle of active learning, rather than individual differences in the learner, support this view. Kolb attempted to improve the original LSI in 1985 and this, too was criticised by Loo (1999). Loo used Confirmatory Factor Analysis to analyse the items within the inventory and failed to support Kolb's (1985) efforts to improve the original instrument. Loo does, however, support the two bi-polar dimensions as well as the LSI itself as a tool for understanding learning and teaching. Further criticisms have been levelled at Kolb's LSI, in relation to distance learning, by Diaz and Cartnal (1999). They argue that Kolb's LSI is, 'primarily a cognitive learning preference instrument, which does not specifically take into account social preferences that are the key distinction between distance and traditional classrooms' (p131).

So, the evidence suggests that Kolb's LSI, despite the contentious nature of its validity, does have practical relevance. It can assist in understanding the way in which students process information and, despite the claims of Diaz and Cartnal (1999), might be applicable to distance learning settings. The next section will move to the third layer of Curry's Onion Model.

Approaches to studying

Approaches to studying represent the third layer of the onion. Included under the heading of approaches to study are those approaches that can be mediated by learning strategies (Curry, 1983). Learning styles and strategies can be modified by external constraints, such as situational variables and aspects of curriculum design (e.g. induction to learning, guidance, design of learning materials, and assignment completion). These factors impact on students' motivation to study which, in turn, influences their approach to learning and learning strategy.

Early work on approaches to studying examined the depth with which students approach the learning task. These were divided into deep and surface approaches. Marton and Saljo (1976) define 'surface' learning as occurring when students try to remember as much as possible from a text. 'Deep' learning, which results in higher level outcomes, occurs when students attempt to de-structure and restructure knowledge, so that the material is related to their own construct system (Morgan *et al*, 1982). The relationship of approaches to studying to curriculum design, referred to above, is illustrated by the work of Trigwell *et al* (1997). This showed relations between teachers' approaches to teaching and student learning. Students, who adopted significantly deeper approaches to learning than their colleagues, were more often taught by teachers who adopted approaches to teaching that were more orientated towards students and to changing their conceptions. The students of teachers, who described their teaching in terms of transmitting knowledge, tended to have surface approaches to learning. This typifies how learning characteristics towards the outer layer of the onion are affected by factors outside of the individual. Marton and Saljo's theories were developed further around concepts of motives and strategies (Entwistle, 1979; 1981; Biggs, 1993). Hence, it was also assumed that a relationship might exist between motivation to study, the strategy arising from the motivation, and the level of learning resulting from the strategy adopted.

Biggs (1993) and Entwistle (1979; 1981) share similar views on motives and strategies. Both argue that deep, surface and strategic approaches are determined by students' motivations and intentions (Murray-Harvey, 1994). Motivations include interest in the subject, fear of failure, and competition. Intentions include the desire to fulfil assessment requirements. Thus, students who are motivated by extrinsic factors, such as qualifications, are more likely to engage in surface learning. On the other hand, students who are motivated by intrinsic factors, such as a desire to master difficult subject matter, are more likely to achieve deep learning. In satisfying their motivations and intentions, individuals adopt specific learning strategies, such as reproducing material or searching for meaning. For example, students who have a strong desire to seek new knowledge and gain satisfaction from learning, (motive) would read widely, applying a new skill (strategy) and would best be described as possessing a deep approach to *learning* (Murray-Harvey, 1994).

Different approaches to *learning* (deep, surface, and strategic) have also been defined from factor analysis studies (see *Table 2.5*).

Table 2.5: Descriptions of three different approaches to learning

Approach to learning	Description
Deep approaches to learning	An intention to understand
	Relating and organising ideas
	The use of evidence and logic
	Active interest
	Search for meaning (Entwistle, 1988; Entwistle and Tait, 1995; Sadler-Smith, 1997:54)
Surface approach to learning	Intention to reproduce
	Reliance on memory
	Passive learning
	Fear of failure
	Difficulty in making sense
	Unrelatedness
	Concern about coping (Entwistle and Tait, 1995; Sadler-Smith, 1997:54
Strategic approach to learning	Study organisation.
	Time management
	Intention to excel
	Control of conditions of study (Entwistle and Tait, 1995; Sadler-Smith, 1997: 54; Richardson, 1992: 38)

As can be seen in *Table 2.5*, students who are most successful in distance learning are likely to use either a deep or strategic approach. The strategic approach is similar to the achieving approach (Entwistle and Ramsden, 1983), which is characterised by competition and ego enhancement, resulting in strategies that maximise time organisation and coverage of syllabus (Chit-Kwong and Kit-Tai, 1996: 76). Although there seems to be general agreement that these three approaches exist, Kember and Leung (1998) dispute this. They carried out a study of 4843 students at the University of Hong Kong using Ramsden and Entwistle's (1981) Approaches to Study Inventory (ASI). Their findings suggest that the strategic/achieving dimension is not a third category, but an additional dimension that can be present with both meaning and reproducing orientations.

Other research into these approaches to study has particular relevance to distance learning. Harper and Kember (1986) researched approaches to study in distance learning compared to class-based study, using the 'Approaches to Studying Inventory' (ASI) (Ramsden and Entwistle, 1981). From 779 completed questionnaires (a 71% response rate), they found that the ASI is valid for use with distance learning students. Jones and Kember (1994) also found that surface learners rely heavily on lectures to set the boundaries for their learning, while students with deep approaches to learning have been shown to be more receptive to self-learning packages than students with surface approaches (Jones and Kember, 1994). Their findings also revealed that approaches to study differ with age. Age differences include the fact that older students tend to be less syllabus-bound, and display learning characteristics associated with higher education. They conclude that older students might 'have learned to assess evidence and relate ideas through their family and work experiences' (p220). However, although older students have not been shown to engage in surface learning, those who do so might be quite vulnerable. As Thorpe points out, adult students working alone may continue for a long time with surface approaches that may frustrate their progress (Thorpe, 1987). This might be particularly problematic at the beginning of a distance learning experience, as new students often believe that learning is about remembering facts and ideas (Taylor and Morgan, 1984).

Although the ASI has proved to be a popular measure of student approaches to study, Waugh (1999) has recently proposed an alternative measurement model. Waugh developed earlier work using a Rasch (1980) analysis to revise the ASI to include 40 *attitude* items and 40 corresponding *behaviour* items (Waugh and Addison, 1998). From these items, five orientations to study were developed—a deep approach, a surface approach, a strategic approach, clarity of direction in studying, and academic self-confidence towards studying. The ten *attitude* items of the strategic approach demonstrated that students found it easy to aim to ensure, *prior* to studying, that they would find conditions that would allow them to get on with their work. The corresponding *behaviour* items, however, revealed that students found it much harder in behaviour than in attitude, to keep their minds on the study task. This same problem occurred in both the deep approach and the academic self-confidence orientation. In relation to the deep approach, students indicated that they set out to understand meaning within the text, but then had difficulty in doing so. The academic self-confidence orientation was characterised by students finding it easy to expect to have a good understanding of subjects and to achieve high standards, but more difficult to achieve this in practice. Waugh concluded that attitudes are easier than behaviours and that the Rasch model helps to explain how behaviours are influenced by attitudes.

The work on approaches to study reveals its significance in helping to understand how students' motivations, as well as external influences, affect the level of learning achieved. It also demonstrates differences between how students expect to approach their study and the actual practice of doing so. These findings have particular salience for distance learning, as students take full responsibility for the way in which they approach their learning, with external constraints in home life having more influence than class-based activities. Approaches to study are, therefore, closely connected to the outside world. The next section will move still closer to external stimuli at the outer layer of Curry's (1983) Onion Model.

Learning preference

The final, outer layer, of the onion refers to learning preferences. Sadler-Smith (1996: 54) defines a learning preference as:

> *'. . . an individual's propensity to choose or express a liking for a particular instructional technique or combination of techniques'.*

Riding and Rayner (1998) consider learning preferences to be crucial because they are an important part of strategy development.

Early work on learning preferences includes that of Canfield and Lafferty (1974) and Canfield (1980), who conceptualised learning preferences by identifying a model comprising four conditions and four modes of learning. Canfield and Lafferty's Learning Styles Inventory (1974) includes four conditions of learning (need for: affiliation with peers, structure, achievement and eminence); four content areas (preference for working with: numbers, words, inanimate objects, people); and four modes of learning (listening, reading, iconic media, direct experience).

The instrument was field-tested on pre-vocational and professional students. According to Canfield and Lafferty (1974), both nursing and physical therapy students expressed significantly stronger needs for organisation and direct experience than did other students studied. Since these groups are likely to include a high number of women, it is pertinent to consider the findings of one of the largest studies of Canfield and Lafferty's LSI in health professionals. Payton *et al* (1979) measured the learning style preferences of over 1000 physical therapy students representing 40.8% of the population from 42 schools. Mean scores indicate that these students preferred working closely and personally with the instructor, for work to be logical and organised, with specific details of assignment requirements, and to work with people, listen and gain direct experience. Physical therapy students dislike independent action, working alone, competing with others or working with numbers or words; nor do they wish the teacher to be the authority figure. Some of these findings are supported by Merritt's (1983) study of non-traditional learners, who prefer the learning environment and methods used in formal settings.

Students' preferences for certain teaching strategies were also the subject of Ostmoe *et al*'s (1984) research of nursing students. Their preferences included: lectures, demonstrations, required reading, course syllabus, films, and case studies. None of the strategies were 'never preferred' and only one strategy, correspondence study, was 'seldom preferred'. They concluded that Baccalaureate nursing students prefer learning strategies that are traditional, teacher-directed and highly organised, while preference for more innovative strategies decreases as students progress through the undergraduate programme. Since these groups comprise predominantly women, they may well typify the preferences of women distance learners.

As with approaches to study, discussed in the last section, research into learning preferences becomes particularly significant when related to student attainment. In assessing student attainment, Hunter (1980) used the Canfield and Lafferty LSI to measure the learning style preferences of over 300 students in three colleges and 15 courses, and compared results to scores on a Student Rating of Instruction instrument, as well as four levels of achievement (A, B, C, D). The findings indicated that A grade students preferred learning modes of listening, direct experience, organisation and detail, while rejecting reading and independence. Average (C grade) students prefer affiliation and independence, while rejecting organisation and detail. Hunter concluded that, if instruction, mode, and content were guided by consumer preference, instruction would probably be 'structured, non-competitive, dependent, authoritative, non-quantitative, people orientated, listening, little reading, and direct experience' (p83).

Some of these modes and conditions are typical of distance education: structure, non-competitive, people-orientated and, to some extent, direct experience. It is interesting that the characteristics associated with distance education are more appropriate to the C grade student than the A grade student. For example, independence is preferred by C grade students, but rejected by A grade students. A grade students also reject reading (a necessary component of distance education) in favour of listening, which is less frequent in distance education. Hunter's findings may, of course, reflect the preferred learning styles of younger students (student age was not indicated in his research) who have not developed adult styles of learning.

It would appear that Canfield and Lafferty's LSI does seem to have some value in establishing student learning preferences, and its use should enable students to consider whether distance learning is a suitable mode of study. Riechmann and Grasha (1974), however, offer an alternative model of learning preferences to that of Canfield and Lafferty. They identified three types of learner, reflecting learning preferences as follows:

- dependent learners, who prefer teacher-directed, highly structured programmes, with explicit assignments set and assessed by the teacher
- collaborative learners, who prefer discussion, group assignments and social interaction
- independent learners, who prefer to exercise an influence on the content and structure of the learning programmes with the teacher as a resource.

Sadler-Smith (1997), using a Learning Preference Inventory, found that dependent learners, as well as preferring teacher-directed, highly structured programmes, with explicit assignments set and assessed by the teacher, also favour lectures and tutorial/surgeries. Dependent learners, therefore, may have difficulty with distance learning study unless lectures and group tutorials are also provided. Collaborative learners prefer discussion, group assignments and social interaction, which is matched with collaborative methods of role-play, discussion groups and business games (Sadler-Smith, 1997). Collaborative learners, too, might dislike distance learning as a method of instruction. Independent learners prefer to exercise an influence on the content and structure of the learning programmes with the teacher as a resource and are, therefore, well matched to open/distance/flexible learning (Sadler-Smith, 1997).

Much of the work on learning preferences indicates students' desire for structure within materials, with clear direction from tutors. Such theories illustrate two factors:

a) the need to diagnose student learning preferences at the commencement of study so that the appropriate mode of study can be selected; and

b) the need to design distance learning curricular in such a way that sufficient guidance is provided for students.

Summary

This chapter has considered a variety of theories of learning style, strategy, and approaches to learning and learning preferences. Each theory can be readily applied to each individual's own learning situation and provides insights into the advantages of different styles, as well as the problems that students adopting such styles are likely to encounter in distance learning study.

It is important to acknowledge, however, that, although individual characteristics of learning are an important influence on the process and outcome of learning, the learning process is also affected by many other factors. In distance learning situations, much learning takes place in the home environment, and this fact alone creates challenges arising from the need to prioritise between study and home-related activities. These tensions will be explored further in *Chapters 3* and *4*.

Reflection

Consider whether your own style, strategy, approach to learning, and learning preferences mirror any of those discussed in this chapter. Then consider whether you would like to develop alternative styles or approaches to learning. If you would like to adapt your learning style, what strategies would you need to employ to enable you to do this?

Practical activity

- Make a list of the *main* characteristics of your learning style or approach to learning
- State what changes, if any, you would like to make
- List any activities that you would need to engage in, in order to bring these changes about.

References

Biggs JB (1993) What do inventories of students' learning processes really measure? A theoretical review and clarification. *Br J Educat Psychol* **63**: 3–19

Busato VV, Prins FJ, Elshout JJ, Hamaker C (1998) Learning styles: a cross-sectional and longitudinal study in higher education. *Br J Educat Psychol* **68**: 427–41

Canfield A, Lafferty J (1974) *Learning Style Inventory.* M I Experimental Learning Methods, Plymouth

Canfield AA (1980) *Learning Styles Inventory: Manual,* 2nd edn. Humantics MediaAnn, Arbor

Carlson B, Keane P, Martin JB (1979) R&D organisations as learning systems. In: Kolb D, Rubin I, McIntyre J (eds). *Organisational Psychology: A Book of Readings.* Prentice-Hall, Englewood Cliffs, NJ

Carnwell R (1996) The challenge of distance education for community nurses: Managing the learning process through student empowerment. In: Oliver P (ed). *The Management of Educational Change—A Case Study Approach.* Arena, Aldershot, Hants: 83–104

Chit-Kwong K, Kit-Tai H (1996) Students' achievement goals and approaches in learning: The relationship between emphasis on self-improvement and thorough understanding. *Res Educ* **55**: 74–85

Cooper R (1977) Learning styles and staff development. *J Nat Ass Staff Dev* **37**: 38–46

Curry L (1983) *An Organisation of Learning Styles and Theory Constructs.* ERIC Doc 235: 185

Diaz DP, Cartnal RB (1999) Students' learning styles in two classes: Online distance learning and equivalent on-campus. *Coll Teach* **47**(4): 130–35

Entwistle NJ (1979) *Motivation, Styles of Learning and the Academic Environment.* The University of Edinburgh: ERIC Document Reproduction Service, No ED 190 636, Edinburgh

Entwistle NJ (1981) *Styles of Learning and Teaching.* John Wiley and Son, New York

Entwistle NJ, Ramsden P (1983) *Understanding Student Learning.* Croom Helm, London

Entwistle NJ (1988) Motivational factors in students' approaches to learning. In: Schmeck RR (ed). *Learning Strategies and Learning Styles.* Plenum Press, New York

Entwistle NJ, Tait H (1995) *The Revised Approaches to Study Inventory.* University of Edinburgh: Centre for Research on Learning and Instruction, Edinburgh

Flannery DD (1993) Global and analytic ways of processing information. *New Dir Adult Contin Educ* **59**: 15–24

Freedman RD, Stumpf SA (1978) What can one learn from the learning style inventory? *Acad Man J* **21**(2): 275–82

Gee DG (1990) *The Impact of Students' Preferred Learning Style Variables in a Distance Education Course: A Case Study.* Eastern New Mexico University: ERIC Document Reproduction Service No. ED 358 836, Portales

Grigerenko EL, Sternberg RJ (1995) Thinking styles. In: Saklofske DH, Zeidner AM (eds). *International Handbook of Personality and Intelligence.* Plenum Press, New York: 205–30

Harper G, Kember D (1986) Approaches to study of distance education students. *Br J Educat Technol* **3**(17): 212–21

Hunsaker JS (1981) The experiential learning model and the learning style inventory: An assessment of current findings. *J Experient Learn Sim* **2**: 145–52

Hunter WE (1980) Relationships between learning styles, grades, and students ratings of instruction. *Community/Jr Coll Res Q* **5**: 73–84

James WB, Gardner DL (1995) *Learning Styles: Implications for Distance Learning.* (ERIC Document Reproduction Service No. EJ 514 356). Jossey-Bass Publishers, California

Jones AE (1997) Reflection-impulsivity and Wholist-analytic: Two fledglings? ... or is R-I a cuckoo? *Educat Psychol* **17**(1 and 2): 65–77

Jones A, Kember D (1994) Approaches to learning and student acceptance of self-study packages. *Educ Train Inst* **1**(2): 93–7

Kagan J, Rosman BL, Day D, Albert J, Philips W (1964) Information processing in the child: Significance of analytic and reflective attitudes. *Psycholog Mon* **78**: 1

Kember D, Leung DYP (1998) The dimensionality of approaches to learning: An investigation with confirmatory factor analysis on the structure of the SPQ and LPQ. *Br J Educat Psychol* **68**: 395–407

Kevin RC, Liberty PG (1975) *Student's Personality, Attitude and Learning Styles as Predictors of Performance in an Undergraduate Organic Chemistry Course using Computer-based Education.* Educational Resources Information Centre, ERIC Document ED 115 209, USA

Kolb DA. (1973) *On Management and the Learning Process.* Working Paper. Institute of Technology, Massachusetts

Kolb DA. (1976) *Learning Style Inventory Self Scoring Test and Implementation Booklet.* McBer & Company, Boston

Kolb DA (1985) *Learning Style Inventory and Technical Manual.* McBer & Company, Boston, MA

Le Cornu A (1999) Learning styles, gender and age as influential issues amongst students of theology. *J Belief Val* **20**(1): 110–14

Lockitt B (1999) Individual learning styles and resource based learning. *Learn Resource J* **15**(1): 4–10

Loo R (1999) Confirmatory factor analyses of Kolb's learning style inventory (LSI-1985). *Br J Educat Psychol* **69**: 213–19

Marton F, Saljo R (1976) On qualitative differences in learning II: Outcome as a function of the learner's perception of the task. *Br J Educat Psychol* **46**: 115–27

Merritt SL (1983) Learning style preferences of Baccalaureate nursing students. *Nurs Res* **32**(6): 367–72

Morgan A, Taylor E, Gibbs G (1982) Variations in students' approaches to studying. *Br J Educ Technol* **2**(13): 107–13

Murray-Harvey R (1994) Learning styles and approaches to learning: Distinguishing between concepts and instruments. *Br J Educat Psychol* **64**: 373–88

Ostmoe PM, van Hoozer HL, Scheffel AL, Crowell CM (1984) Learning style preferences and selection of learning strategies: Consideration and implications for nurse educators. *J Nurs Educ* **23**(1): 27–30

Pask G (1976) Styles and strategies of learning. *Br J Educat Psychol* **46** : 128–48

Pask G, Scott BCE (1972) Learning strategies and individual competence. *Int J Man-Mach Stud* **4**: 212–53

Payton OD, Hueter AE, Mcdonald ME (1979) Learning style preferences of physical therapy students in the United States. *Physical Ther* **59**: 147–52

Plovnick MS (1975) Primary care career choices and medical students learning styles. *J Med Educ* **50**: 849–55

Ramsden P, Entwistle NJ (1981) Effects of academic departments in students' approaches to studying. *Br J Educat Psychol* **51**: 368–83

Rasch G (1980) *Probabilistic Models for Some Intelligence and Attainment Tests* (expanded edition). University of Chicago Press, Chicago

Reifle S, Edwards A (1975) *C-BE Education Instruments: A Descriptive Report.* Educational Resources Information Centre, ERIC Document ED 115 210, USA

Richardson JTE (1992) A critical evaluation of a short form of the approaches to studying inventory. *Psychol Teach Rev* **1**(1): 34–45

Riding RJ (1991) *Cognitive Styles Analysis: User Manual.* Learning and Training Technology, Birmingham

Riding RJ (1997) On the nature of cognitive style. *Educat Psychol* **17**(1&2): 29–49

Riding RJ, Rayner S (1998) *Cognitive Styles and Learning Strategies: Understanding Style Differences in Learning and Behaviour.* David Fulton Publishers, London

Riechmann SW, Grasha AF (1974) A rational approach to developing and assessing the construct validity of a student learning styles scale instrument. *J Psychol* **87**: 213–23

Sadler-Smith E (1996) 'Learning style': A holistic approach. *J Eur Indust Train* **20**(8): 29–36

Sadler-Smith E (1997) 'Learning style': frameworks and instruments. *Educat Psychol* **17**(1&2): 51–63

Schmeck RR, ed (1988) *Styles and Strategies of Learning.* Plenum, New York

Sternberg RJ (1988) Mental self-government: A theory of intellectual styles and their development. *Hum Dev* **31**: 197–224

Sternberg RJ (1990) Thinking styles: Keys to understanding human performance. *Phi Delta Kappan* **71**: 366–71

Sternberg RJ (1996) Styles of thinking. In: Baltes PB, Staudinger UM (eds). *Interactive Minds: Lifespan Perspectives on the Social Foundation of Cognition.* Cambridge University Press, Cambridge: 347–65

Tait H, Entwistle N (1996) Identifying students at risk through ineffective study strategies. *High Educ* **31**: 97–116

Taylor E, Morgan A (1984) *Students' Open University Careers, Study Methods Group Report No 14,* IET. Open University, Milton Keynes

Tennant M (1988) *Psychology and Adult Learning.* Routledge, London

Thorpe M (1987) Adult learners in open learning. In: Thorpe M, Grugeon D (eds). *Open Learning for Adults.* Longman Open Learning. Harlow, Essex: 71–82

Trigwell K, Prosser M, Lyons F (1997) Defining good teaching: Relations between teachers' approaches to teaching and student learning. Paper presented at: *The Conference of the European Association of Learning and Instruction,* August, Athens, Greece

Vermetten YJ, Vermunt JD, Lodewijks HG (1999) A longitudinal perspective on learning strategies in higher education: Different viewpoints towards development. *Br J Educat Psychol* **69**: 221–42

Vermunt JD (1994) *Inventory of Learning Styles in Higher Education; Scoring Key for the Inventory of Learning Styles in Higher Education.* Tilburg University, Department of Educational Psychology

Vermunt JD (1996) Metacognitive, cognitive and affective aspects of learning styles and strategies: A phenomenographic analysis. *High Educ* **31**: 25–50

Vermunt JD (1998) The regulation of constructive learning processes. *Br J Educat Psychol* **68**: 149–71

Waugh RF, Addison PA (1998) A Rasch measurement model analysis of the revised approaches to studying inventory. *Br J Educat Psychol* **68**: 95–112

Waugh RF (1999) Approaches to studying for students in higher education: A Rasch measurement model analysis. *Br J Educat Psychol* **69**: 63–79

Witkin HA, Moore C, Goodenough D, Cox P (1977) Field-dependent and field-independent cognitive styles and their educational implications. *Rev Educat Res* **47**: 1–64

Wunderlick R, Gjierdl CL (1978) Another look at learning style inventory and medical career choice. *J Med Educ* **53**: 45–54

3
Approaches to study in distance learning

This chapter describes a research study in which three approaches to study emerged from the data. The three approaches to study are explained in detail, drawing on literature reviewed in *Chapter* 2. The study involved interviews of twenty female registered nurses studying distance learning modules, to either gain a diploma or sufficient credits to access a community health degree.

The sample

The twenty students were selected from a previous survey (n=120), in which 96 students responded to a questionnaire. The questionnaire, as well as asking about students' experience of distance learning, also invited them to participate in an interview. Over half agreed and provided contact details. These were divided into two groups representing the two courses studied, 'Research Awareness' and 'Access' modules. There were ten students in each group. Each group was then divided (according to their responses to the questionnaire) into those who were positive about their distance learning experience, those who were negative, and those who were ambivalent. Twenty students were then selected for interview in a way that ensured that a minimum of three students from each category was represented. This type of purposeful sampling ensures that participants will be selected who will provide useful insights that address the research question. This method is particularly appropriate for qualitative research (Clifford, 1997).

The interview

Ethnographic interviews were conducted, each lasting approximately 90 minutes. The goal of the interview was to research the topic from the perspective of the interviewee, and to understand how and why she came to have a particular perspective (King, 1994). A quite detailed, but flexible interview guide was used, as suggested by King. The relationship between researcher and interviewee was also an important part of the research process. Rather than a distraction from the research, the interviewees were seen as participants, actively shaping the course of the interview, rather than passively responding to it (King, 1994). Thus, a low degree of structure was imposed by the researcher, with mainly open questions focussing on sequences of events and specific situations identified by each participant (Kvale, 1983). The interview addressed issues, such as: how students typically approach their reading; learning preferences; preferred structure of materials; previous experience of study; preferences for dialogue and tutorial needs; and motivation to study.

Critical ethnography (Thomas, 1993) was also used during the interviews and the interpretation of the data. Critical ethnographers attempt to uncover socio-structural explanations for people's behaviour. In this case, the focus of interest was on how society and culture might have influenced the perception of the distance learning experience for these women, who were working full-time while studying. Typical of the questions a critical ethnographer asks might be, 'Are nurses pressurised by society to engage in further study, and how does the nursing culture influence their experience of learning'? The critical ethnographer, however, has to ensure that her/his own understanding is accurate and, therefore, the researcher's understanding is interrogated by reflecting the researcher's interpretation back to the participant. An example of this would be:

Participant: One of the good things about doing the course when I did, was that several other nurses had already completed it. Everyone seemed to either be doing it, or was going to do it in the near future. So the support of others was really important.

Interviewer: Are you saying that there was pressure in nursing generally to become more academically qualified?

Participant: No, that's not what I meant really, that wasn't the reason I did it, but I did get the benefit of the support from others who had done it before.

This interaction demonstrates the importance of the researcher interrogating her/his own understanding when using critical ethnography. In trying to find cultural explanations for the participant's views (i.e. a cultural shift in nursing towards higher academic qualifications), it is easy to misinterpret what the participant actually meant.

How the interviews were analysed

Once the interviews were complete, they were transcribed verbatim, then summarised to make the data more manageable (Miles and Huberman, 1994). The next stage used the principles of open and axial coding suggested in grounded theory (Strauss and Corbin, 1990). Open coding involves a line-by-line analysis, asking questions such as 'What is this? What does it represent? The answers to such questions can then be given conceptual labels. Later, categories within concepts can be developed and these categories can be assigned properties. Before discussing the labels imposed by the researcher, concepts, categories and properties will be defined.

Concepts are defined as 'conceptual labels placed in discrete happenings, events, and other instances of phenomena' (Strauss and Corbin, 1990: 61). An example of a conceptual label from this research is 'approach to study'. This label was applied as it accurately described the phenomena of *how* students went about their learning. The distance learning situation could, therefore, be described as the discrete happening or event.

Categories are 'discovered when concepts are compared against one another and appear to pertain to a similar phenomenon' (Strauss and Corbin, 1990: 61). An example of the development of a category was the comparison of the concept of 'approach to study' between different students. This gave rise to three categories—systematic wader, speedy focusser and global dipper.

Properties are defined as 'attributes or characteristics along a continuum' (Strauss and Corbin, 1990: 61). An example of a property would be all the characteristics of each of the three categories within the concept of 'approach to study'.

During open coding, data is broken up into smaller components. The purpose of axial coding, therefore, is to reassemble this fractured data. Axial coding involves relating categories 'to their subcategories to form more precise and complete explanations of phenomena' (Strauss and Corbin, 1998: 124). An example of this can be seen in the concept 'orientation to study', which included four categories describing students' orientation to study—vocational, academic, personal development, and compensation. A vocational orientation was typified by responses indicating the need to study modules in order to access a degree, as indicated in the following quote:

> *'It was work-related and I needed the degree to get on personally and I needed these modules to get on the degree.... You were pushed I suppose, with vocational things you are pushed. You have to be more determined, more of an attitude that you must succeed ... I suppose in some ways I didn't enjoy it as much knowing that I had to do it*[7]*'.*

This quote illustrates an important link between a 'vocational orientation', and the concept of motivation. Thus, such links demonstrate the reassembling of data to form explanatory links involved in axial coding. A more detailed account of this coding process follows.

Development of the concept of approaches to study, its categories and properties

Concept one: approach to study

Reading and re-reading of the interview transcripts revealed that students seemed to study at a different 'pace', and furthermore, if given a text to read, different students would approach their reading of the text in different ways. Some would start at the beginning, reading everything, others would dip in and out. Some would want advice from other people, while others did not feel the need for this. This phenomenon was given the conceptual label of 'approach to study'. Further analysis revealed that three categories seemed to typify the different approaches:

- systematic waders
- speedy-focussers
- global dippers.

The systematic wader

Typically, 'systematic waders' progressed through the materials in a systematic and rigorous manner, taking few short cuts, characterised by the comment from one student:

> *'I started at the start with this* [the module] *and an A4 pad of paper and a pen. I might have scanned the contents page just to see what it was about. I would probably have read the introduction because I didn't know what was expected of me, and I remember writing 'chapter one, what is sociology', and I made notes under each heading*[10]*.'*

Another systematic wader commented:

> *'I read all the way through everything ... I don't skim read, I sit and read it rigorously ... it's always been that way, if I do something, I want to do it properly, I don't half do things*[4]*.'*

This comment also suggests that systematic waders take a *maximalist* approach to learning. When asked if she would read the off-prints at the recommended time, she answered: 'Yes, I always do as I'm told'[4]. This suggests that systematic waders do not select their reading according to its *relevance*, but read as instructed instead.

This *maximalist* approach was also highlighted in another comment:

> *'I would just plough all the way through it from beginning to end. I like repetitive things, so I might test myself by doing the activities. Then I'd actually sit down with the information in front of me to see if I could recall anything I was supposed to have learned. If there was, say, three answers I would write those three answers down again, and if I felt I hadn't learned it and it was important to me, I'd go back and read it again, or do it again*[2]*.'*

Some comments suggested that systematic-wading typifies the approach to study of inexperienced students, who go on to adopt other patterns as they gain experience. Some students, for example, had changed from being systematic waders to being more selective (possibly speedy-focussed) since completing a degree course, as in the following two comments:

> *'I used to take a big deep breath and start going through it, I think now ... whereas I used to go through from the start, now I would probably go through the off-prints first. I would have started at page one and gone through it, now I might have a quick look at the introduction to see what was in, but I would definitely go to the off-prints and read some of these first before tackling the book . . . The way I've changed is that I try to check through the introductions, because I'd discovered that there can be quite a bit in the introduction that will give me an insight. Where I would have just ploughed in before, now I'd be a bit more selective, so instead of getting bogged down thinking I've got to read pages and pages, I tend to try to be selective[9].'*

> *'I tend to plod through . . . because I'd feel that I'd got to do it all . . . I'm reading what I think I've got to read, not what I want to read. I've done further study since and now I'd skim read, but I did this very much the hard way ... Boxes and summaries are helpful. If I was using these now, I would read those first, before the text . . . If I'd understood what was expected of me I wouldn't have got so bogged down with the actual practicalities of reading these . . .[11].'*

The speedy-focusser

Speedy-focussed learners would focus very quickly on what was required and would adopt a very efficient and effective learning strategy, as in the following quote:

> *'I'd probably speed read it, and something like a questionnaire, I'd probably completely ignore it, I would just speed read it... Possibly what I might do, depending on how interesting these are, is look at the main chapter bits, reading the first bits of each one[6].'*

This participant seemed to be flexible in her approach to reading, but also to approach it as a holist, rather than a serialist. When discussing the types of activity she liked to engage in, another speedy-focussed student commented:

'I would list those in my head. If it involved writing things down, I probably wouldn't bother. I'd just move on to the next one... Inductive reasoning, again I could do this in my head, so I'd probably just list them in my head. I'd probably take a short cut there as well. You can see how quickly I'd work through . . . Case studies, they usually take longer, I would probably just pass over those, unless it was something that was particularly pertinent to the end result. With distance learning, the end result [passing the assignment] *is just the be all and end all*[5]*.'*

For this student, time seemed to be a factor that influenced her speedy-focussed approach to studying. Referring to case study type activities, she remarked:

'If it's going to take five minutes I'll do it, if it's going to take an hour I won't[5]*.'*

This student went on the describe practical activities and comprehension activities as time-consuming, causing her to miss them, but would engage in an activity relating theory to practice because:

'. . . that could be quite easily and quickly done. I would probably do that because it doesn't involve writing anything down[5]*.'*

However, she was also a serialist learner when the situation seemed appropriate:

'I decided what I was going to do [for the assignment], *then I read it* [psychology module] *from cover to cover in relation to the assignment that I'd got to do. So to me, again, everything concentrates on the end result—the assignment*[5]*.'*

Selective note taking also seemed typical of speedy-focussed learning:

'I'd write 'page 13'. Then I'd write what I was looking for in page 13, e.g. 'good quote on quantitative'. Then another example later on of something else ... I may put a star by it so that when I come back to look for it, I can just look down the reference list, rather than reading through[5]*.'*

The global dipper

Global dipper learners would study in a disorganised fashion, moving to and fro within the materials, but, unlike speedy-focussed learners, it would appear to be without a pre-determined plan, as in the following quote:

> *'I actually read the off-print first, then the contents page, then picked out the things that looked more interesting and read what I wanted to read, and took notes of what I felt was interesting to me. A quarter of the way through the course I thought, 'This isn't for me', but it was something I had to do for the diploma. So I didn't go through it chronologically, and just turned to the sections and took notes from all of them, but not in any particular order[15].'*

Global dipping was also the only approach to study that was characterised by reference to what other students did. It appeared that reference to other students supported and perhaps, therefore, excused their own study behaviours.

> *'I think I did like most people. We got to about book 4 or 5 and maybe 6 and then did no more of the books, and if you needed some explanation you would flick through the next few books and see if there was an answer there that would help you. But if you're thinking 'what am I going to do, how an I going to set this out, I've looked at so and so's research proposal and I've looked at so and so's proposal and they are different, she uses these words and she uses these words'... I switched off from them and went on to other books[16].'*

Another student started with the first book because:

> *'I didn't know how much I'd got to read. . . I read the first one all through, and then thought 'I don't know whether I'm going to be able to read the whole lot'. So I started to pick up the topics, where I thought it would be nice to read, and easier quick reading, and then I started being selective and looking at different things that I could do and might be useful to me. . . I discussed it with the other girls, I said 'do we have to read all these books, I'm getting a bit bored'. . . I asked a friend what books to read, and she recommended Polit and Hungler, and I could understand that better than going through all of these. . . The distance learn-*

ing materials get more complicated because some of them tell you to imagine this and do that. . . The textbook gives you ideas, they just write it in and you just read it. . . I know they've got a lot of guides to tell you how to do it, but I find it difficult to keep going back to this and thinking about how it's used and applied to this theory or that theory[13]*.'*

Another student also started logically, but then changed her approach due to dissatisfaction:

'I tried to read it logically the first time, but didn't understand so started to dip in and out, got totally confused and went and got a book on research, then came back and read it systematically[17]*.'*

When asked if she read all the books in order, she replied:

'No, I read them out of order ... I felt that the books weren't covering all the nursing situations, it was just ward-based, which was annoying ... and there is nothing allied to the community ... and you think 'oh, that's got nothing to do with me' which makes it difficult ... I went to another book, and a second book. I communicated with other students on the course who were having similar problems[17]*.'*

These quotes illustrate how global-dippers search for answers from a variety of sources, including alternative text books and other students, and then return to the text, still searching for understanding. The third quote also indicates that, unlike systematic waders (who make no selection according to the relevance of the reading), global dippers appreciate materials that are relevant to their work situation.

The characteristics of the three approaches to study, identified within the above quotes, are described as 'properties' and are listed in *Table 3.1*. Numbers in brackets refer to interpretation of student quotes identified in the preceding analysis.

Table 3.1: Properties of the three different approaches to study

Category	Properties
Systematic wader	Is obedient and inexperienced at study (9) Is rigorous, 'ploughs through' systematically(2) Gets 'bogged down', feels a sense of obligation (9,11) Makes copious notes and memorises to understand (10) Engages in serialist learning (4)
Speedy focusser	Takes short cuts, engages in thinking not note taking (5) Reads selectively (5,6) Prioritises around the assignment and time constraints (6) Speed reads, uses margin notes (6) Engages in flexible holist learning (5,6)
Global dipper	Flicks through, and struggles with content (15, 13) Needs guidance, searches for answers, seeks advice and compares self with other students (16,17) Resorts to other texts in desperation (16,17) Engages in minimalist learning, using flexible serialist and holist approach (15,13, 16) Views knowledge as 'given'

It is interesting to note that global dippers consult other books when they experience difficulty. This is typical of an 'application-directed' learner (Vermunt, 1996) in which learning style is concerned with usefulness of learning content and realising personal goals. Application-directed learners, however, make schemes and resort to an analytic strategy, whereas global dippers seem to rely on advice from other people to build up a complete picture. The schemes and analytic strategy adopted by application-directed learners seem more typical of speedy-focussers. Speedy-focussers also seem to be impulsive in their study (Kagan *et al*, 1964) by reaching decisions quickly after a brief review of opinions and this, in fact, might be a deliberate strategy, as suggested by Jones (1997).

Global dippers, having a 'with-people' orientation, also seem to be field dependent (Witkin *et al*, 1977), whereas systematic waders, being able to work in a solitary manner seem to be field independent. Systematic waders also appear to have an internal scope of self-government, since they are happy to work on their own (Sternberg, 1990). They also seem to be *reproduction-directed*, and this is characterised by selecting the main parts of the materials by underlining (Vermunt,

1996), and resembles Entwistle's (1988) reproducing orientation (Vermetten *et al*, 1999). As indicated in *Chapter 2*, such students follow the advice of course writers in distinguishing major and minor points, and have little difficulty making selections. They appear to adopt a serialist approach to learning (Pask, 1976) by learning sequentially, step-by-step, part by part, studying every topic separately. They also resemble the executive function of self-government (Sternberg, 1990) by consulting no other sources than the course materials and following instructions. Reproductive learners seldom reflect on their learning or find out for themselves the cause of their difficulties and this, too, seems to resemble systematic waders.

Another important difference, between systematic waders and global dippers, is the way in which they view knowledge. View of knowledge was, therefore, the next concept to be labelled.

Concept two—view of knowledge

View of knowledge was divided into two categories—'know--ledge given' and 'knowledge sought'. Students categorised as 'knowledge given' were more concerned with passing the assignment, rather than mastering the knowledge contained within the package. Mastering knowledge contained within the package would typify the response of students who view knowledge as something to be 'sought'. Students categorised as 'knowledge given' also completed assignments in a manner that enabled them to complete the task rather than deepen their understanding. Knowledge as 'given' was, therefore, characterised by a desire to be supplied with knowledge, rather than taking responsibility for seeking and developing one's own knowledge. This seemed to be related to students' reasons for studying, as in the following examples:

> *'I resented having to do it, because I was doing it as a means to an end. I wasn't thinking 'oh I'll enjoy that', I was doing it because I had to do it to get on the course[12].'*

> *'I wasn't really there to learn, I was there to get those credits to get on that course. So if I learnt anything along the way it was a bonus. Whereas if you go on a particular course, e.g. the Health Visitor course, I went there to 'yes' qualify at the end, which you*

> *could argue is the most important thing, but I wanted to learn the profession and the theory that went with it. I was keen to learn on the Health Visitor course, but keen to pass on the distance learning*[5]*.'*

By comparison, students categorised as viewing knowledge as sought, commented:

> *'If I get a reading list, and I go away and look, a) it makes me look and I also find other things that are interesting. And b) if it's a research module, you really ought to be out there, not having it fed to you on a plate, but looking for articles*[19]*.'*

> *'I was motivated to pass the assignment, but there is no pleasure in that if you are not mastering the knowledge. The knowledge is what gives you the pleasure to do it. The knowledge is there to get it right. And I wanted to get it right at the end. . . If I get it wrong then I haven't got the knowledge and I wanted to understand that*[8]*.'*

Given these comments and others that were similar, the properties associated with the category of a view of knowledge are as listed in *Table 3.2.*

Table 3.2: Properties associated with view of knowledge

Category	Properties
Knowledge as given	Instrumental motivation (12,5) Importance of the course to career prospects (12,5)
Knowledge as sought	Interest in subject matter for its own sake (19) Self-directedness (19) Mastery of knowledge (8)

Students who view knowledge as 'given' are often vocationally orientated and typify application-directed learners, who do nothing with the materials that do not interest them, viewing knowledge as present only if it can be used (Vermunt, 1996). Viewing knowledge in these different ways assumes that some knowledge is more relevant than other knowledge. Relevance of reading was, therefore, the next concept to be identified

Concept three—relevance of what students read

As noted above, systematic waders and global dippers each referred to the relevance of what they read. Students typically viewed learning as being worthwhile if it was relevant. For systematic waders, relevance was not important in determining their reading, whereas global dippers might reject certain sections of the materials, if these were not relevant to their work situation. Frequent reference, by the participants, to the 'relevance' of the content of distance learning materials led, therefore, to the formulation of the concept of 'relevance of reading'. Relevance to their work situation was, normally, the way in which they appeared to define relevance, as in the example of one student who defined a good learning experience, thus:

> *'We now have a specialist nurse who runs her own course to teach community nurses about leg ulcer care. It's relevant, practical and she sets us a test at the end... It was relevant to the job, direct contact with the tutor, small groups, and relevant to everyday practice[8].'*

For this same student, a bad learning experience was also defined in relation to relevance:

> *'There had been a lot of build up on things that were relevant and it started off badly and was wasting my time[8].'*

This would seem to suggest that learning that is not considered relevant to the students' particular needs may be deemed to be a 'waste of time'. Another student selected the research awareness module because of its relevance:

> *'For me everything's got to be relevant. I did the course because it was relevant, and everything I do has got to be relevant[19].'*

When asked what made her decide not to read some of the modules, she responded: 'relevance to me again[19]'. Thus, relevance appears to be important to students at two different levels: in selection of courses, and selection of reading of materials within the selected course. Indeed, students made varying levels of selection of reading of distance learning materials, and relevance seems to be the main criteria that determines what they read. Thus, five different categories were developed within the concept of relevance, which determine how students select what to read.

Categories of relevance

The first category, 'reading as instructed' suggests that such students make no selection at all, as in one student who remarked that:

> *'I've heard some people say they didn't find them* [the modules] *much value, but if I'm given something I do it. I rarely question it until the end or if it gets really hard going. I'm prepared to give anything a try*[8]*.'*

Another student made a connection between 'reading as instructed' and the philosophy of distance learning:

> *'I'm quite good at distance learning, if I'm supposed to do it I do, so I went through it methodically*[19]*.'*

Reading as instructed seems to suggest an unquestioning approach to reading selection, a sense of optimism, acceptance, being methodical and obedient. These properties appear to overlap with the systematic wader approach to study.

The second category, 'relevance to assignment', highlights the fact that, for some students, relevance to the assignment is the dominant factor that determines their reading:

> *'Given the pressure of time, I still think that if I had all the time in the world and I'd got a question to answer, I'd look at the sections that would give me the answers to the question*[12]*.'*

For another student, interest might drive some of her reading, but relevance to the assignment seemed to take a higher priority:

> *'I might have made some brief sketchy notes on things I was interested in. I might have referenced a book and paragraph on a piece of paper if it was relevant or if I might need it, and that's where the dipping in comes in*[14]*.'*

When asked what it needed to be relevant to, this respondent answered:

> *'...the assignment, the way that I dissected the research, something to tell me how to do it*[14]*.'*

For some students categorised as maximalist learners, relevance to the assignment directed further reading: 'If it was relevant to the assignment, then I'd read it a third time[7]'.

A midwife, categorised as reading what is 'relevant to the assignment and work', commented that:

> *'Some of the psychiatric activities didn't appeal to me and I would probably abbreviate in that situation, just to get through it[20].'*

When asked if she would write things down when doing the activities, she responded:

> *'It depends whether I thought I would need it, because some of them you do. If I had already got my research proposal in mind and I thought it would be beneficial, then I would make notes[20].'*

Relevance to the essay and work was also characterised by the following comment:

> *'I might have read it more than once to try to understand it, then pick out the bits that I want to remember, or that I thought were important. . . Maybe when I say I want to remember, I think of things that might be useful in the future, or for doing the assignment[10].'*

Other students extend their definition of relevance to include the essay and interest, as in the following comment:

> *'I was conscious of what the assignment was at the end, and I was probably skipping through things that I thought wouldn't help with an assignment. . . unless I found it quite interesting, in which case I would read it for enjoyment[10].'*

One student explained how she shared her more interesting content with her work colleagues:

> *'When I was reading psychology, people would say 'what are you reading' and I would say what I was just reading about, and they would say 'oh that sounds really interesting' and it would often start conversations and people would say 'oh I think that'[1].'*

It was sometimes difficult to distinguish 'relevance to the assignment' from other categories of relevance, for example, work or self-interest. Students may, initially, appear to be motivated to read for interest or relevance to work, but frequently mentioned the assignment as a factor that determined their reading when questioned further. The only exception to this appeared to be students who read because they were instructed to do so. These students would cover the relevant reading for the assignment, during the natural progression of their reading. The properties of the different categories of relevance, identified from these quotes, can be seen in *Table 3.3.*

Table 3.3: Properties of the different categories of relevance

Category	Properties
Reading as instructed	Reading with unquestioning acceptance (8) Possessing a sense of optimism (8) Being methodical and obedient (19)
Relevance to assignment	Searching for clues to answer the assignment (12) Dipping in the materials (14) Skipping through the materials (10)
Relevance to work	Reading what is useful to work (20)
Interest	Reading for enjoyment, and enjoy sharing with others (1)

As these properties developed, links became clear between different concepts and categories, as is typical of axial coding. Links exist, for example, between the categories of 'relevance', the three categories reflecting the three approaches to study, and serialist or holist learning. Holists or flexible holists appear to prioritise their work in relation to its interest and relevance to the assignment. Such students have similarities with Sternberg's (1990) judicial function of self-government, in that they select their reading according to its practical relevance, and search for relations between the subject matter and the reality to which it refers. In this way, such students will sometimes read for interest, if the content captures their imagination during their initial dipping into the materials. If their imagination is not captured by the content, they will focus in on the specific content that is relevant to the assignment. These characteristics confirm Flannery's (1993) belief that global information processes must be connected to what people value in their own subjective worlds, or it will be discarded as unimportant. Schmeck's (1988) suggestion that such learners scan in order to form overall impressions and are more intuitive and impulsive than analytics, also seems to be confirmed by these findings.

The link with approaches to study occurs with students who tend to wade through the materials (and also tend to be serialist learners). Generally, these students do not prioritise and read as instructed. According to Pask and Scott (1972), serialists attempt to build understanding, focussing on details, logical relationships between argument and evidence, and on operations taken strictly in a linear sequence (see *Chapter 2*).

These findings, relating to how students prioritise within the materials, seem to suggest different levels of commitment. Thus, this became the next concept to be labelled so that it could be explored in more detail.

Concept four—commitment

As indicated above, some students seemed to become more committed to their learning than others. Some students, for example, read everything, while others read selectively. This led to the concept of 'commitment' being identified. Commitment, which refers to the amount of time students devote to their studies, was categorised as either maximalist or minimalist learning. Maximalist learning was characterised by reading either more than the normal requirement, or during periods when reading would not normally take place, as in one student who took the modules on holiday:

> *'Some of the things were very interesting and I even took the books on holiday*[8]*.'*

For other students, maximalist learning directed them to further reading:

> *'If they recommended that I read a certain book or chapter from somewhere else, I'd try and search for it in the mean time, but I'd skip that if I couldn't find it and come back to it later*[7]*.'*

When asked if she would ever take short cuts, this same student commented that:

> *'No, well it's there for a reason, and you're instructed to read it... I missed some of the questions in the exercises because I wanted to crack on with the theory. But most of those sections, of the psychology one I did, I just went through it because it was there for a reason*[7]*.'*

These comments suggest a link between 'maximalist learning' and 'reading as instructed' (labelled as relevance in the above discussion). Such comments, however, also imply that students may actually prioritise while not recognising that they are doing so. Instead, they possibly classify their reading as 'instructed' because this is what they have come to expect from their previous learning. Maximalist learners also appear to engage with the materials and gain satisfaction from completing and understanding the course, as in the following comment:

> *'But I'm quite a logical worker and I like to feel that I've gone through it so that I can say I've done the course and understand it*[18]*.'*

This student adopted a serialist approach, completed 75% of the materials, found the materials to be well-designed, liked closed materials (i.e. well-structured) and would find her own way through them. By contrast, students defined as minimalist learners did the minimum of reading:

> *'When I'm doing a task, research etc., I won't sit around for ages wading through stuff. I'm lazy, actually, I save time by just getting it done*[6]*.'*

Although this student described this attribute as lazy, it could also be a definable attribute of speedy-focussed studying. This student also went on to identify other examples of so-called laziness:

> *'There were bits where you were encouraged to go off and read a bit more about it. Looking back I could have put an awful lot more thought and time and consideration and thinking into it, rather than saying 'oh I know that, I know that …'*[6]*.'*

When asked if she did anything to try to understand she replied:

> *'No, I was possibly lazy, at that stage. I just wanted to get on the course. There was loads of other stuff going on* [domestic circumstances] *and at the time it wasn't related to what I was doing* [her job]*. So it really was just a case of get this down on paper, get it handed in and passed and then you can start the course*[6]*.'*

She later said that she did very few activities, since she either skipped them or cheated. Although this student defined herself as lazy, her comments do reveal the importance of 'relevance to work' as a factor that determines reading, while also suggesting that students described as minimalist learners might be prioritising between a variety of work and domestic commitments. Other students also illustrated these points:

> *'But when you're trying to fit it in with everyday life and work, you don't put the full effort in*[16]*.'*

> *'I didn't discipline myself enough to go back over points that I didn't understand.... Because I was quite frightened when I first started it, I found it difficult to motivate myself to start with. I became more motivated when I started to do things that were of relevance to my work environment*[9]*.'*

This same student went on to say:

> *'I have achieved a lot, when I think about it now, because without doing this, we wouldn't be doing some of the things we're doing within the practice*[9]*.'*

Another student defined laziness in terms of self-discipline and application:

> *'Perhaps I'm not a good candidate for distance learning because I'm lazy and don't apply myself unless I have to do something... If there had been no assignments attached I don't know whether I would have done it... I'm not disciplined. I use it* [distance learning] *when it's relevant and I can't get on a course*[2]*.'*

This student was also categorised as a systematic wader who appreciated internal dialogue. Minimalist learning could also be explained in terms of energy preservation, as indicated in the following comment, in which the student was discussing the merits of internal dialogue (i.e. the author entering into a dialogue with the reader by highlighting different arguments, or providing instructions):

> *'There's very little energy expended in flicking through those. Someone else has done all the thinking and I just have to identify something*[11]*.'*

The distinguishing properties between maximalist and minimalist learning and are listed in *Table 3.4*.

Table 3.4: Properties of maximalist and minimalist learning

Category	Properties
Maximalist learners	Portray a maximalist interest (8) Are obedient in selection of reading (7) Are committed to study (18).
Minimalist learners	Experience pressure of time (6) Make priorities between learning and other commitments (6,9) Need self discipline and motivation (6) Need to preserve energy (9,2) Select reading according to its relevance (16,2)

What seems to be emerging from student commitment to distance learning, is that some students devote more time to learning than others, and this may possibly result in a different level of outcome.The approaches used by minimalist learners could reflect the desire for older students to be less syllabus-bound and to assess evidence quickly, based on their work experience (Harper and Kember, 1986), or it could reflect a surface approach to learning (Marton and Saljo, 1976). Certainly, students with deep approaches to learning have been shown to be more receptive to self-learning packages than students with surface approaches, and it could be that maximalist learners are demonstrating this characteristic (Jones and Kember, 1994).

Summary

What has become evident, so far, is that students approach their study in different ways and seem to have different levels of commitment to study. What then became interesting was whether these findings had implications for curriculum design. The interview transcripts were scrutinised to discover whether students with different approaches to study also had different preferences for the way in which materials are designed, as well as their type and amount of interaction with other people. These factors will be explored in the next chapter. Before beginning the next chapter, readers may wish to engage in the following reflection and practical activity.

Reflection

Consider whether your own experiences of learning bear any similarities with students' experiences discussed in this chapter.

Practical activity

- Identify which, if any, of the concepts and categories applies most aptly to your learning experiences
- State what you can learn from the students' experiences and how you can apply this to your own learning
- Return to the practical activity at the end of *Chapter 2* and consider whether your list of activities should be amended in the light of the above.

References

Clifford C (1997) *Nursing and Health Care Research: A Skills-based Introduction* (2nd edn). Prentice Hall, London

Entwistle NJ (1988) Motivational factors in students' approaches to learning. In: Schmeck RR (1988) *Learning Strategies and Learning Styles.* Plenum Press, New York

Flannery DD (1993) Global and analytic ways of processing information. *New Direct Adult Contin Educ* **59**: 15–24

Harper G, Kember D (1986) Approaches to study of distance education students. *Br J Educat Technol* **3**(17): 212–21

Jones AE (1997) Reflection-impulsivity and Wholist-analytic: two fledglings? ... or is R-I a cuckoo? *Educat Psychol* **17**(1&2): 65–77

Jones A, Kember D (1994) Approaches to learning and student acceptance of self-study packages. *Educ Train Inst* **1**(2): 93–7

Kagan J, Rosman BL, Day D, Albert J, Philips W (1964) Information processing in the child: Significance of analytic and reflective attitudes. *Psycholog Mon* **78**: 1

King N (1994)) The qualitative research interview. In: Cassell C, Symon G (1994) *Qualitative Methods in Organisational Research: A Practical Guide.* Sage, London: 14–36

Kvale S (1983) The qualitative research interview: A phenomenological and a hermeneutical mode of understanding. *J Phenomenolog Psychol* **14**: 171–96

Marton F, Saljo R (1976) On qualitative differences in learning II: Outcome as a function of the learner's perception of the task.*Br J Educat Psychol* **46**: 115–27

Miles MB, Huberman AM (1994) *Qualitative Data Analysis—An Expanded Sourcebook,* (2nd edn.). Sage, Newbury Park, CA
Pask G, Scott BCE (1972) Learning strategies and individual competence. *Int J Man-Mach Stud* **4**: 212–53
Pask G (1976) Styles and strategies of learning. *Br J Educat Psychol* **46**: 128–48
Schmeck RR, ed (1988) *Styles and Strategies of Learning.* Plenum, New York
Schmeck, RR (1998) *Learning Strategies and Learning Styles.* Plenum Press, New York
Strauss A, Corbin J (1990) *Basics of Qualitative Research: Grounded Theory Procedures and Techniques.* Sage, London
Strauss A, Corbin J (1998) *Basics of Qualitative Research: Grounded Theory Procedures and Techniques,* (2nd edn.). Sage, London
Sternberg RJ (1990) Thinking styles: Keys to understanding human performance. *Phi Delta Kappa* **71**: 366–71
Thomas J (1993) *Doing Critical Ethnography.* Sage, London
Vermetten YJ, Vermunt JD, Lodewijks HG (1999) A longitudinal perspective on learning strategies in higher education: Different viewpoints towards development. *Br J Educat Psychol* **69**: 221–42
Vermunt JD (1996) Metacognitive, cognitive and affective aspects of learning styles and strategies: A phenomenographic analysis. *High Educ* **31**: 25–50
Witkin HA, Moore C, Goodenough D, Cox P (1977) Field-dependent and field-independent cognitive styles and their educational implications. *Rev Educat Res* **47**: 1–64

4
Support and guidance for distance learning

Introduction

The interview responses discussed in *Chapter 3* indicated that different approaches to study adopted by students might have important implications for curriculum design. Curriculum design includes a variety of factors designed to facilitate learning, such as the design of the learning materials to which students are exposed and the support mechanisms to assist students to gain maximum benefit from their learning. Thus, further concepts relating to these issues were developed and are presented in this chapter. For the purpose of this chapter, these concepts are grouped into four sections as follows:

- Guidance through text design
- Student approaches to study and related guidance and support needs
- Guidance through tutorial provision
- Support needs of women distance learners

Section one—guidance through text design

Following the literature on text design (Bernard and Lundgren, 1994; Hartley, 1988a; 1988b), text materials can be defined as being either *high* in structure or *low* in structure. Highly structured materials are characterised by specific guidance regarding the timing and order of reading and use of materials; prescribed activities, and in-text exercises, and all resources and readings being contained within the package. Materials low in structure adopt a more flexible approach, with suggested readings that students are required to select from and find for themselves, with less reliance on timed activities. The literature, together with student responses to previous questions, led to the labelling of the concept of 'structure of materials'.

Concept five—structure of materials

During the interview, participants were given one of the texts that they had studied and were asked questions about their preferences in relation to text structure and other features they found helpful. The range of responses resulted in the development of categories relating to openness of materials. Three categories were: closed, neither open nor closed, and open. Typical responses generating a 'closed' category were:

> *'For me, that* [objectives with checklists] *would be quite good.... I wouldn't feel that people were trying to check up on me. I'd think they were trying to keep me on track and make sure I was still focussed, because that's one of the great disadvantages of distance learning. I like the idea of someone on my back ... to ensure that I'm still doing the work... it keeps me on track[9].'*

This quote illustrates links between 'direction' from objectives, external checking of progress, and keeping 'on track', developed later in this section. Another student, preferring closed materials, highlighted the need for structure:

> *'I've done one distance learning course before for an asthma diploma, which was very structured, and there was a video with it as well to help you along with the study and a big pack of things that you could work through... It was almost as if there was somebody next to you all the time telling you what to do, which way to do it, and I felt much more at home with that. We had two days at a training centre ... an introduction to what was in the course and what would be expected of us.... There were lots of practical things to do ... case studies, and speaking to patients[4].'*

One student[6] who liked closed materials made the link between structure and 'self help' by stating that she would not contact a tutor if advised to do so by a checklist at the end of a section, but would contact colleagues and peers instead. If she did not understand set objectives, a checklist at the end of each section would help because:

> *'It doesn't give you that excuse to skip over it. You can miss all this out and no one is ever going to know and you can pretend to yourself that you did do it. But if you've got that checklist at the end and you've got to put your ticks in it, it's there to see that you've not done it. I need a bit of discipline probably. I need to prove to myself that I've done it. I'm a very listy kind of person[6].'*

Students whose preferences suggested neither closed nor open materials needed less structural cues, but still needed the text to provide some direction.

> *'I wouldn't need all that* [advance organiser] *and in fact this probably goes into too much detail, e.g., the block is broken up into six chapters. You can see that in the contents page anyway[10].'*

This student did, however, appreciate other structural features, such as objectives with checklists although not at the end of each section.

A student categorised as preferring open materials commented that a well-structured text would be achieved by:

> *'... breaking it down into sections and actually titling those sections ... having a list of relevant reference material. I don't know whether that's necessary* [suggested timings]. *The actual activities tend to take different times anyway. I'd ignore it* [a learner profile] *... just more work[2].'*

Another quote generating an 'open' category was in response to a question concerning use of objectives and checklists:

> *'It's something else you've got to fill in. I think because you've got progress boxes, activities and questions you've already got enough cross-references[15].'*

This same participant also expressed a dislike of advance organisers with timings.

The different structural preferences exhibited by students reflect different degrees of need for direction within the materials. Properties relating to the different categories of material structure are presented in *Table 4.1.*

Table 4.1 Properties of open and closed materials

Category	Properties
Closed	Practical tasks, videos, face-to-face, case studies, discipline, external monitoring, direction, timings, regular checklists, practical examples, opportunities for discussion (4, 9, 6)
Neither open nor closed	Infrequent objectives, checklists, few advance organisers (10)
Open	Titled sub-sections, list of relevant reading, cartoons and pictures, progress boxes, summaries, activities, questions, no objectives, no checklists, no organisers (2, 15)

It would seem, then, that features that distinguish the preference for closed or open materials are as follows:

- the need for direction through the materials
- the use of structural cues
- the need for guidance from an external source such as face-to-face introductions and opportunities for discussion.

The need for direction through materials confirms the work on learning preferences (Canfield and Lafferty, 1974; Merritt, 1983; Payton *et al*, 1979), indicating that students need structure within materials with clear direction from tutors. The use of materials to provide direction is also an important means of providing support for students—a concept that will be considered further in the next section. Much of the literature on support for distance learners, for example, focusses on the use of materials. Examples include: use of text devices, such as illustrations in learning materials (Martens *et al*, 1996), technological innovation (Harrison, 1997; Kommers *et al*, 1998), and provision of information (Johnson, 1999) to support learning. The preference for face-to-face introductions and built in opportunities for discussion is also a feature of external dialogue, the next concept to be identified within curriculum design.

Concept six—dialogue

Dialogue is an interesting concept to curriculum design, as it can be incorporated, not only into text design, but also within tutorial support (to be discussed later). The use of dialogue differs from, but co-exists with, structure of materials. Evans and Nation (1989:37) define dialogue as involving the idea:

> *'that humans in communication are engaged actively in the making and exchange of meanings, it is not merely about the transmission of messages.'*

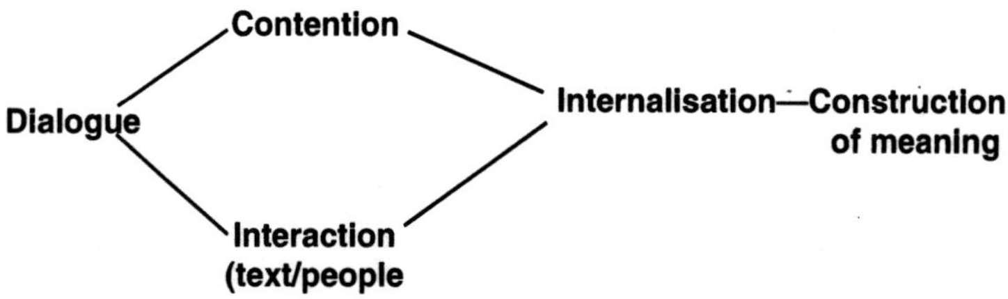

Figure 4.1: Dialogue and the construction of meaning (reproduced with kind permission from Hargreaves D (1978) *Sociological Interpretations*. Studies in Education, Driffield)

As *Figure 4.1* suggests, dialogue is a means through which students are introduced to contention and dissension in relation to various concepts and theories. It is through the exchange of meanings involved in dialogue that students internalise the meaning of concepts. The results of this research suggest that different types of dialogue are important to students. Dialogue can take place both *within* the package (internal) and *externally* to the package.

Internal dialogue occurs in two different forms. Firstly, authors communicate with the reader using internal dialogue. This involves more than the 'transmission of messages' (Evans and Nation, 1989), since it introduces contention and dissension in order to enable students to construct meaning. Secondly, internal dialogue can involve additional materials to the text, thus providing assignment guidance and helping students to 'map' their progress. The need identified by Access students for better explanation, clear assessment guidelines, and highly structured materials illustrates this point. It is probable, therefore, that dialogue is used more rigorously in highly structured material. The desire for structure (internal dialogue) could result in increased dependence on the package. Nevertheless, dialogue can enhance independence and power of students through tutor support (Moore, 1990).

It is the dialogue offered through tutor support that is defined here as 'external' dialogue. External dialogue can be initiated both between the student and tutor, and between the students themselves. It is these latter types of dialogue that are representative of the need for *support*, which will be discussed later in this chapter.

The two types of dialogue, internal and external, were identified prior to the interviews. They were defined and explained to participants in order for them to specify their preferences. Internal dialogue was explained in terms of an author of materials attempting to engage the student interactively. An example given by the researcher during each interview is as follows:

- The author explains three theories, theory A, B and C, and asks you to consider which is the most legitimate. The author then goes on to say that most people prefer theory A and then points out why. The author then goes on to explain that people often think that theory B is more legitimate, but if you felt that theory C was the best one, then you could have been thinking in a certain way.

Students who were in favour of internal dialogue could see various advantages:

> *'I think it would be useful because it's almost like having a tutor there. But you'd have to be disciplined not to read the answers... You'd have something concrete to look at and reassure yourself that you were going in the right direction. It would give you something to bring to the tutorial as well*[19]*'.*

> *'You come across a situation and they introduce different theories and you can reflect at that time and think 'oh yes it's that one'. And then have your own little thoughts and discussion with the author in the book, by them saying 'if you chose that theory it was this', and then you instantly think of a scenario in your head. So to me having that there, reading it and then think-*

ing it up yourself at the time, is better than loads of thinking when you see them [tutors] *and say 'now what was that theory?' You know you're going to have to make points, whereas if you just look at it and make decisions yourself by reflecting, that's better*[3].'

One student would respond to internal dialogue, but would prefer it:

'*. . . if there were three* [theories] *and two were wrong, and you could pick out which one was right. There are rewards if you get them right, and there's very little energy expended in flicking through those. Someone else has done all the thinking and I just have to identify something*[11].'

Some students appreciated the value of internal dialogue, but did not feel that this would be sufficient to compensate for external dialogue. Such students were, therefore, coded as preferring both types of dialogue (internal and external). One student, for example, expressed a lack of confidence that would drive her to seek guidance from someone, although she felt that it might satisfy a need for feedback, initially:

'But if there was a big question mark against what theory I'd come up with, ...I might start thinking ...why have I chosen theory A when most people choose theory B'. But then I might get a bit worried and think 'am I grasping this the same as everybody else'. So I might need someone to speak to[9].'

For another student, the need for internal or external dialogue depended on the content of the module. This student had studied both sociology and psychology access modules, and had enjoyed psychology but not sociology. She explained that internal dialogue:

'Involves you ...so that it crystallises it in your mind to some degree... You don't have to interact with the text if it's just information written and it's not requiring you to apply yourself to it... As I'm reading the psychology module, I'm thinking to myself, 'do I agree with that or not', and I found with sociology I didn't know whether I agreed with it or not. I didn't know what the opposing view was. It wasn't set out in such a way that they would say, 'this is one view on it and this is another view', so

> *that you could actually decide what you thought... I don't think it can completely substitute for that* [external dialogue]. *It's not until other people have an opinion and you think, 'I would never have thought about that' ...so I think there's a limit to how far you can broaden your thoughts on something when you've only got your own view of things to use*[1]*.'*

This student also made a link between submitting checklists to a tutor as a means of monitoring progress and the need for guidance:

> *'A lot of preparation to start off with and that has to be with a person you'd associate as the link person who you can go to if you've got problems or need support, and then some sort of systematic time period. It's very loose, so you think 'am I taking too long over this'. It says you can work at your own pace, but you don't know whether the pace you're working at is an average kind of pace, very laborious or whether you're doing it in a very superficial way*[1]*.'*

A link between external dialogue and closed materials can also be seen in the comments of student 1. Some students expressed a definite preference for external dialogue:

> *'For me, external. I'd get more out of it, because I would tend to think 'oh yes', if it was something I was reading saying this theory or that theory, I would say 'oh yes I agree with that'. Whereas, if I was talking to someone who is likely to ask me a question and why I thought that, I think I would think far more deeply, rather than just skim over it*[12]*.'*

For another student, external dialogue would only be of more benefit in its capacity to provide feedback on writing style:

> *'As far as doing the content of the two pieces of work, yes, fine. But I think it was the style that you're writing in, or your grammar, or sentence construction, and things like that, that's what students need feedback on*[18]*.'*

This would suggest links between dialogue, material structure, need for guidance, and view of knowledge, which are explored in more detail later. Properties associated with the different categories of dialogue can be seen in *Table 4.2*.

Table 4.2: Properties of different types of dialogue

Category	Properties
Internal dialogue	Provides sense of tutor presence, discipline, concrete reassurance, direction and rewards (19, 11) Used to facilitate a tutorial (19) Encourages reflection (3)
External dialogue	Provides external discipline for minimalist learners (12) Provides feedback on writing style for maximalist learners (18)
Both	Assists confidence building (9) Provides assistance in understanding materials (1) Encourages deeper learning and broadens thinking through discussion (1)

As can be seen from the above discussion, students with different approaches to study might also have different needs of dialogue. Furthermore, dialogue seemed to be crucial in providing guidance and support to students.

Section two—student approaches to study and related guidance and support needs

Student responses to the need for different types of dialogue raised issues relating to the need for guidance, as well as the need for support. These two concepts appeared to be related to each other, as well as to the concept of dialogue. In order to understand the relationships between these concepts, however, it was first necessary to define each concept separately and to identify its categories. As guidance seemed to be closely allied to dialogue, this was identified next.

Concept seven—guidance

The concept of guidance reflected the need of some students to be directed to what to read, external dialogue often being viewed as the source of this information. Students were either categorised as needing 'guidance through the materials', or being able to 'find own way', depending on whether they expressed a need for guidance or not. Students who were defined as being able to find their own way were those who either needed no guidance of any kind, or needed minimal guidance, normally associated with the assignment, but were quite happy to find their own way through the materials. One student pointed out the need to be motivated:

> *'There's no point thinking this is something where you can sit in a few lectures and not participate, because you're not going to get anywhere. This is something you really have to do yourself. You have to be motivated to do it, and it's your responsibility to realise that you have to understand what you're learning, or you're not going to get anything out of it*[18]*.'*

However, this same student did need guidance concerning the assignment about half way through the module. Another student, needing minimal guidance concerning the assignment, and who had previously spent four years studying with the Open University, commented that:

> *'It took a long time from reading that* [the text] *to being able to answer the questions and do projects. There wasn't a lot of guidance between the two. You had to really think hard, and sometimes it was off at a tangent to the question, and you hoped that the answer would become clear.... I think there could have been more* [guidance].... *We were left to the question and that was it*[7]*.'*

A sense of 'hope' was also echoed by another student who said:

> *'I must say, with distance learning you have to get on with it and hope for the best and just hope that you're going in the right direction... Apart from the fact that I do have confidence in my own ability, I don't have a problem with learning... it wasn't the doing of it that was a problem, it was the principle of distance learning*[20]*.'*

Another student, who was happy to find her own way through the materials, commented that:

> *'I went along on the night, that was fine, everyone in the library was very nice and explained where everything was, how everything was referenced, and that they would help. I didn't have any problem with that at all*[18]*.'*

Another student felt that the materials should provide the guidance needed:

'They guide you through it, rather than someone phoning you up and saying 'have you done chapter two yet?', or even someone saying 'how are you finding it'[6]?'

These comments provide an interesting comparison with those that follow. Students who needed to be guided through the materials were more vociferous with their comments. Their responses suggested the need for two different types of guidance: *introduction* to the module, and *guidance throughout* the learning process.

The manner in which they were introduced to the materials was very important to them, and this applied equally to the two types of modules. For the research awareness module, students were sent a study guide in advance, which explained the nature of the module. They were also sent joining instructions to attend an introductory evening tutorial from 6–8 p.m. At the introductory evening, they enrolled on the module and were introduced to the nature of distance learning and the module content. They were also introduced to the library services during which they collected the entire pack of twelve books. Students reacted to this experience in a variety of ways, feeling daunted being a common response, as illustrated by the comment of one student:

'I think to apply to do a distance learning module and to be given 12 books and to go away and read them, is quite daunting… We had a brief introduction to research and were told not to worry about it and it's pretty easy, go to the library and collect your books... I wished I'd never gone, I just thought 'this is going to be a six month struggle'… We did have a study guide [in advance] *and looking at that I thought it was going to be enjoyable, until I got to the university[17].'*

Another student echoed these feelings:

'The first night I didn't have a clue what I was doing. That really struck me, I thought 'oh my goodness what have I done'. I always thought when you did distance learning, you could do it in your own time... I thought I could do it in a year's time. But when I went and they said 'this has got to be finished by December and another lot by February, it struck me that I'd just gone blank... There's a whole lot of books and I thought 'oh my dear,

I've got to read all through these... there's no way, I don't know where I'm starting from'... It would have been nice if we had got a list of things that 'this is what the answer to the question is approximately, much earlier than that night... If there had been a better guide saying which books to read and where to tackle it[13].'

Another student expressed similar views:

'You were given about 12 books and never shown how you should go through them. You were carted down to the library, signed in 'here's your pile of books, off you go'... Then you read them and the first two or three, you think 'this isn't too bad'. Then you get to a stage when you're not really understanding what you're reading, so you skip it[16].'

Students offered solutions to this problem, such as being given the books in stages:

'Rather than saying 'here's the first three, go and pace yourself'... I think if you had completion dates [at different stages built into the package] *it encourages you to get the work done[17].'*

One student suggested a briefing day before the course starts:

'Saying 'this is distance learning, this is what is expected of you', before you sign on the dotted line. 'This is the way forward for tutorials' and brainstorm what you want from tutorials[15].'

Another student commented on the nature of research as a difficult subject:

'It was way above us and we didn't know anything about it... I think if you can get over the awe of the word 'research'... which it is to a lot of people ... then you can look at it in a different way[9].'

For this student a 'starter pack' would have been beneficial:

'Just the format of what the course was going to be. How it was going to evolve with the groups. What was expected of you at the end of it, and just give you some idea, a bit of an introduction to research ... something to perhaps put my mind at rest, put me at ease, because I found it quite scary to start off with[9].'

For one student, samples of what was required would have been helpful:

'If they included a sample of 'this is what is good to put in a literature review, you need to take this as a set book'... a sample of it, then we would have known what it was[13].'

Students, who were studying the Access modules, expressed similar concerns, but had experienced a different type of introduction. They were introduced to the modules on an individual basis rather than through a large introductory tutorial. Because these students commenced their studies when they wished to and because no group tutorials were involved, they made an appointment to attend the university and collect the modules. They were enrolled by an administrator and directed to the library, where the librarian provided the materials. This experience also caused problems of isolation and vulnerability:

'I think I had quite a bad experience of its presentation because the question was given to me by a secretary, with a map of how to get to the library to pick the pack up, and a phone number for tutorial support... I felt very isolated... unsupported... vulnerable really[12].'

'I came on my own for the Access modules and it was the receptionist, so I felt a bit isolated with that, because at the same time you're given the essay, so it was 'here you are'. So I think possibly a tutor spending 5–10 minutes to say 'we're looking at this sort of thing, this is what you work through', it just gives you that back up. But as it happens I just got on with it anyway, but it would have been nice[3].'

One student provided specific advice on how the module should be introduced:

'If you'd had a one-to-one with someone who just talked you through it, said ... 'have you thought about how you are going to do this? What's the purpose of doing it? What do you hope to get out of it?'... Your learning style, and whether you're the sort of person who is going to benefit from a tutorial ... it was very difficult to approach someone you didn't know to discuss something that you didn't really understand or have any feeling about[1].'

A student, later coded as a speedy-focussed learner, studying both an Access and a Research Awareness module without tutorial support, suggested:

> *'A set session, perhaps half way through the package, stating that the students should have reached a certain stage, quite dictatorial really. Because that also gives you an aim to be at that stage by that time, which is quite difficult. With distance learning there isn't a date when it's got to be done by, so if I had not had the incentive to finish in time for the course, I don't think I would ever have done it; and a fairly small tutorial with similar ability students*[5]*.'*

Guidance *throughout* the learning process was also important to some students, and appeared to be linked to a closed structure of materials, and tutors taking an active role. It was interesting that guidance *throughout* the learning process appears to be more problematic for research awareness students who have monthly small group tutorials, than it does for the access students who have no such opportunity. One student, who found difficulty both with the subject of research, and with the distance learning philosophy, stated:

> *'I think there's too much. Reading this you tend to fall asleep half way through, they've crammed too much into it*[17]*.'*

When asked how it could be made less dense she replied:

> *'The only way you could do that is with more tutorial sessions. That's the only way really ... It's nice if you're in a classroom and there's someone there at the front who knows research back to front, and they can initially make you want to do research and to understand it*[17]*.'*

Another student experienced some very negative emotions concerning the first small group tutorial, which took place four weeks into the programme of study.

> *'The first one* [tutorial] *when we went into small tutorial groups was very daunting. We had to do our first assignment, which was a critique and she* [the tutor] *said 'I want to know how you're all getting on' and my colleague and I thought 'we don't know how we're getting on' and we were frightened. We just wanted to run out of the room*[16]*.'*

When asked what she would want from a group tutorial this same student said:

> *'A tutor to chat to each person for ten minutes rather than discussing things in the whole group[16].'*

The data suggests that certain properties can be identified according to various categories of guidance, as in *Table 4.3.*

Table 4.3: Properties of the different need for guidance of different student groups

Category	Properties
Find own way	Thinking hard and tangentially (7) Being experienced at study (7) Being fatalistic (20) Being intrinsically motivated (18,6)
Introductory guidance Research awareness	Feeling daunted and scared by awesome subject matter (16) Perceiving that there is little time for volume of reading (13) Needing a 'staged' approach, and gentle introduction (13,17,15,9)
Introductory guidance Access students	Feeling isolated, vulnerable and unsupported (12,3). Needing face-to-face introduction to personal tutor to facilitate future interaction (1)
Guidance throughout	Experiencing fear (16) Dislike of research jargon (16) Needing instruction on precisely what to read and how precisely to tackle the assignment (16) Needing personal attention from tutor (16,17,5)

The need for guidance exhibited by these students, supports Riechmann and Grasha's (1974) research into learning preferences. In particular, students needing guidance throughout the learning process resemble Sadler-Smith's (1997) dependent and collaborative learners in their need for teacher-directed, highly structured programmes, with explicit assignments, discussion and social interaction.

As indicated above, the concept of guidance is closely linked to the concept of support. Indeed, the very act of providing guidance for students is in itself supportive. Support, however, is more complex than merely receiving guidance at the appropriate time, and this was the next concept identified.

Concept eight—support

The relationship between support and guidance can be seen in Sewart's (1987) argument that group interaction, evident in class-based learning, cannot be replaced by a package, since students' needs are not wholly related to the subject being studied. Sewart seems to imply that other needs, such as support, are a high priority for students. The challenge for distance educators is to enable students to access appropriate support mechanisms (including resources), so that knowledge within packages can be re-constructed into the student's own frame of reference.

Support has also been linked to other important concepts, including independence and power (Garrison and Baynton, 1987; Moore, 1990). This combination of the elements of support, independence, and power enable students to gain control over the learning process (Garrison and Baynton, 1987). These relationships are mediated, however, by communication between the tutor and student.

Three categories of support became evident within the interview data: academic, emotional and practical. Some students needed all three types of support, while others need none at all. Academic support was characterised by one student's appreciation of the responsiveness of her personal tutor when she commented that:

> *'If I'm doing something it's got to have access instantly. There was a particular lecturer at the university at the time who was particularly helpful to me, and him I praise. He acted for me at a particular time straight away. He lived close by, I went to his house, and he didn't help me, but gave me a book that was relevant. It was at the right time and appropriate ... When you're doing this it's got to be instant otherwise you get disheartened[8].'*

This quote also illustrates a link between providing academic support and adopting the passive tutor role of 'being available' (discussed later). The blurring of the distinction between academic support and the tutor role was also seen in the following comments:

'Having the opportunity for an individual tutorial, one or two, because a lot of the time, as long as you have the opportunity there, you just need the reassurance to spend an hour, or perhaps two. Not everyone would take up the offer[19].'

'There needs to be a time that you can say 'if you phone me between 10 and 12, I will be there on the phone'. You might not need it, but knowing that it's there can give you the confidence to carry on[14].'

One student's definition of academic support was to 'sit down with me and tell me where I'm going wrong or what I'd doing right[4]'. This was defined in relation to tutorials and, therefore, this student would also be described as preferring the tutor to take an active, rather than passive role. Properties associated with academic support could be defined as: responsiveness, appropriate information, reassurance, availability of tutor 'just in case', and specific direction from the tutor.

One student defined practical support as help given by doctors with whom she works:

'I went to the doctors at work and said 'help' and they were marvellous. They were very helpful finding BMJs and would help me and show me parts that would be useful. They brought books in from home[4].'

For this student, practical support was closely related to emotional support, which was defined as 'asking for help and getting it[4]'.

Some students defined practical support in relation to the family:

'I got support from the family, the fact that they helped in the house... Not even emotional really, more practical, 'we'll give you this time, I'll do the housework and look after the baby, you do your essay[6].'

Properties relating to the category of practical support could be defined as help with information for assignments, help with housework, and childcare. Emotional support was seen in more abstract, psychological terms, rather than physical:

'Emotional support would come from my family and friends... I'd expect them to keep out of my way when I was doing assignments, and be understanding[2].'

One student explained emotional support in terms of 'the understanding that they knew that this wasn't easy for me, that this was a sacrifice that I was making[14]'. For another student, coping with her frustration seemed more important:

'Sometimes I would say 'I'm sick of this' and threw the papers on the floor, and he [husband] *would pick the papers up and say 'now come on let's start again'. My husband did do his best. All my assignments have drawings and headings and calligraphy. He did all that, he got me the stationery materials. He was my total support[15].'*

One student also made an interesting distinction between academic support and emotional support:

'It would have been emotional support really, because it would have been reassurance as opposed to academic[19].'

Another student expanded on this distinction stating that:

'The big confidence builder comes from your family really, saying 'you can get through this'. In the beginning that's when the tutor gave the confidence and emotional support to crack on with it, saying that it's not as daunting as it looks and you need to pace yourself[7].'

Thus, the properties associated with the category of emotional support can be defined as: creating emotional space and tolerance, cajoling, and providing confidence through reassurance. This type of reassurance can be distinguished from academic reassurance. Academic reassurance is acquired through tutor accessibility, while emotional reassurance provides confidence, but without evidence that the students can succeed. The properties relating to the three types of support are presented in *Table 4.4*.

Table 4.4: Properties of different types of support

Category	Properties
Academic support	Appropriate information (8) Responsiveness, reassurance, availability of tutor (8,19,14)
Practical support	Help with information for assignments (4) Help with housework and child care (6)
Emotional support	Tolerance and creating emotional space (2) Cajoling, providing confidence through reassurance (7,15,19)

The need for support seems to be a salient characteristic of distance learning for women and this is confirmed by other studies as discussed in *Chapter 1* (Pascoe, 1977; Kirkup and von Prummer, 1990; Pym and Atkinson, 1990; Pym, 1992). There is also substantial literature examining support in relation to distance learning (Bailey and Moore, 1989; Lebel, 1989; Vowles, 1990; Simpson, 1993). The concept of support will be discussed further in *Chapter 5*.

The need for guidance and support is also reflected in various concepts, including: the structure of materials, and the need for different types of dialogue. These concepts also link closely to students' preferences for tutorials and the way in which they are conducted by tutors. The role of the tutor in providing guidance is, therefore, fundamental to the process of distance learning.

Section three—guidance through tutorial provision

In distance education, good tutoring is as important as well-designed packages in producing good quality open learning (Bailey, 1992). Perhaps the main difference between the distance education tutor and the face-to-face teacher is the balance between the nature of the tutor-student relationship and the need for content expertise. For face-to-face teachers, content expertise is probably the primary concern, whereas for distance education tutors, the fact that content is contained within course materials frees their time to become 'a genuine, respecting, open person first, and a content expert second' (Burge, 1988:15). Given all the 'unkowns' that create the emotional baggage of life experience, the distance educator can only hope to develop rapport through the provision of support. Support in the form of tutorial provision will also prevent the distance learner from becoming an isolated learner (Kelly, 1987). The distance education tutor is, therefore, a facilitator of information rather than a communicator of information, and this includes enabling students to help each other to solve problems which, in an ordinary class, they would put to their teacher (Perraton, 1985).

The facilitator role creates a dilemma for distance education tutors, who favour student autonomy and yet are unsure of how much to intervene in students' learning. A balance is needed between offering too much support and advice that may be perceived as officiousness, and leaving students to fight for survival (Holmberg, 1989). As Holmberg points out, this is aggravated by the additional family and social commitments involved with being adult students.

The role of the tutor as a facilitator in open learning has been examined by Bailey (1992), who suggests that activities on the teaching-facilitation spectrum can be clustered into four areas: the locus of control; learning methodology; learning context and media; and the curriculum. The first two activities, locus of control and learning methodology, are pertinent to this chapter and will be discussed further below.

Bailey argues that the *locus of control* should pass to the students, who should take responsibility for self-assessment, diagnosing strengths and weakness, formulating study plans and using feedback. Bailey argues that both students and tutors often inherit authoritarian models of learning, which impede distance learners in their attempts to 'turn on to the executive material that meets their goals, and turn off that which does not' (Moore, 1973). This concern is also expressed by Burge (1988) who points out that tutors vary widely in their need for power and control, some knowing no other style for working with learners. Leonard and Jowett (1990) also highlight the fact that some teachers lack confidence in self-direction, and compensate by packing the course with taught theory.

The *learning methodology*, Bailey describes, as creating opportunities for dialogue and negotiation of assignments, thereby facilitating the integration of theory and practice, and development of critical thinking. She believes the learning context shifts from focussing on static elements of knowledge towards the learning process itself. Thus counselling, trouble-shooting, and helping learners manage their learning become roles of the tutor. This notion of 'helping' learners places teachers in distance education in an ancillary, supporting, helping role, to be drawn on by students if they so desire (Moore, 1973). This process of using advice and support helps students to fit new knowledge contained in packages into their own pre-existing intellectual framework, as well as their everyday attitudes and behaviour (Sewart, 1987).

The comments from interviews for this research indicated how important the tutor role was to students. Moreover, students had very definite preferences about the role tutors should adopt, and tutorial preferences became the next concept to be identified.

Concept nine—tutorial preferences

The concept of 'tutorial preferences' included reference to the role that students thought that tutors should adopt during group tutorials, as well as in relation to providing academic support. This gave rise to three categories:

- active tutor, in which students felt that tutors should actively teach the subject in tutorials, or should be active in providing support in between group tutorials
- passive tutor, in which students felt that tutors need not take an active role, but should still *be available* in between tutorials, for example by stating specific periods of availability for telephone tutorials
- self-help, in which students preferred to use self-help groups, either in addition to, or instead of, tutorial support.

Some students preferred all three types of tutorial support, while others preferred just one. These different categories justify further discussion.

Active tutor role

An active tutor role was characterised by the importance that students placed on relationships with tutors. After commenting about general dissatisfactions arising from unavailability of a tutor for tutorials, combined with what she perceived to be disinterest of the same tutor, one student commented:

> *'I wouldn't encourage anyone to do it. I think a lot of it is to do with barriers from relationships with tutors[17].'*

Another student was less critical of the tutor, but still found the relationship problematic:

> *'Over the phone I was made to feel like the student from hell because I didn't understand... I always felt that I had to say 'sorry to bother you but' and I normally had quite a list of questions, because I was eager to learn and it was the first time I'd had distance learning. So I wanted to make sure I was on the right track, and I just felt that I was hogging the tutor's time too much, when really she had done her best with all of us, and the rest of us wanted to go home[15].'*

This student went on to discuss how the tutor should take an active role in tutorials by asking students what they had learned, and then guiding them to what they need to read before the next tutorial, rather than what she considered to be unstructured:

> *'What problems have you got? ... and you always get into groups. The yappers, I do wish that the tutors would say shut up[15].'*

From this student's point of view, an element of control is also included in an active tutor role. In a later comment relating to how the distance learning experience could be improved, she commented that 'the odd phone call of encouragement, that would be super[15]', indicating the proactive nature of the tutor's role.

Other students felt that the tutor should take an active role in tutorials by explaining what was required in the assignment, such as:

> *'What is needed in the assignment and what would make it better. Presentation as well, ... then towards the end, if there's any questions[13].'*

Properties of the category 'active tutor role' can, therefore, be defined in terms of: student/tutor relationships, directed reading, control, proactive contact with students, and specific assignment guidance. An interesting overlap occurs between the properties associated with an active tutor role and properties associated with the need for guidance.

Passive tutor

The passive tutor role was closely allied to academic support, within another concept labelled as 'support'. The blurring of the distinction between academic support and the tutor role was also seen in the following comments:

> *'Possibly having the opportunity for an individual tutorial, one or two, because a lot of the time, as long as you have the opportunity there, you just need the reassurance to spend an hour, just one, or perhaps two, not everyone would take up the offer[19].'*

> *'There needs to be a time that you can say 'if you phone me between 10 and 12, I will be there on the phone'. You might not need it, but knowing that it's there can give you the confidence to carry on[14].'*

Properties associated with a passive tutor role could be defined as: responsiveness, reassurance, and availability of a tutor 'just in case'.

Self-help

The third group of students under the heading of tutorial preferences preferred to use self-help groups rather than either an active or passive tutor. One such student commented that when she met with her fellow distance learning students on commencing the community health degree:

> *'We said that if the tutors could have put us in touch with other people doing it, we would have got together[6].'*

Other students felt that this would be totally inappropriate, as indicated by the following comments:

> *'I only wanted it* [dialogue] *with tutors on the course. I didn't want it with other students. That's why I like distance learning, I wasn't competing with anyone else, I did it for me[8].'*

> *'Deep down I feel that I'm in a competitive situation. I tend to find that other students shake my confidence... one-to-one with*

a tutor is probably the best way. I don't trust my fellow students to be giving me the input[11]*.'*

'I don't think so; they're confused as well, they can get you more confused, so it would be more beneficial to talk to someone who can guide you, like a tutor[19]*.'*

It seems that to be successful in a self-help group, students must have confidence in their own abilities, as well as those of their fellow students. There appears to be a link between the need to be guided through materials, the preference for an active tutor and a desire not to engage in self-help groups. These sub-categories proved not to be mutually exclusive, some students indicating a need for both passive and active tutor roles, as well as making use of self-help groups if available. Properties related to the different sub-categories of tutor roles can be seen in *Table 4.5*.

Table 4.5: Properties of the different preferences for tutor roles

Category	Properties
Active tutor role	Value good relationship between students and tutors (15,17) Need tutor to take control in tutorials (13,15) Prefer the tutor to be proactive in contacting students (15) Need directed reading and specific assignment guidance (13)
Passive tutor role	Need tutor to be available 'just in case' (14, 19) Value responsiveness and reassurance from tutor (19)
Self-help groups	Need to have confidence in own abilities, as well as those of fellow students (11,19) Need to avoid competition (8,11)

The above analysis identified several important points about students with different approaches to study, in that they:

- approach their reading in different ways
- have varying degrees of commitment to learning
- prefer different types of structure within learning materials
- need different types and levels of guidance
- need different types of support outside of tutorials
- need different types of interaction with tutors and other students

- prefer different types of tutorial support.

The findings began to raise questions about what impact these factors have on the learning process, as well as the outcome of learning. Some students, for example, often referred to the way in which they organised their learning, and it appeared that being organised might be linked to other personal characteristics discussed above. The concept of 'organisation' was generated in order to explore this further.

Concept ten—organisation

The concept of 'organisation' arose from discussions with students about the way in which they approached the preparation of their assignment. The concept was divided into organised, semi-organised and disorganised. These categories illustrate how students manage time and space during assignment production. Organised students were typically goal-orientated and tended to use time not normally associated with study, as indicated by the following comment:

> *'I set myself goals and would do it to that goal, e.g. by the end of this week I will have done... I never have extensions. I just do it. A Bank Holiday was devoted to it. It's not as structured as saying so many hours a night, but the outcomes have got to be achieved[8].'*

In comparison, a semi-organised approach would be partly dictated by shift patterns, these being common among the sample. As one student pointed out:

> *'Because I work shifts, it's hard to study during the week because I'm up at 3.30 a.m. one week and the next week I don't get home until 11 p.m. ...so I tend to do all my studying at the weekends. I'm an early studier, so I used to get up early at the weekends and then study, and then everyone was up later, so it was mostly weekends—perhaps taking a bit to work and reading behind the subject in the meantime[7].'*

Typically, students using a semi-organised approach would attempt to do some studying at work:

> *'I'd need to know exactly where I was going with it... I tend to carry it around with me, and I take it to work, and as I thought of something I'd just scribble it in. I didn't do it* [referring to study timetable] *on a regular basis. I had to decide when my husband was off for the day so that he would take my son out for the whole day. You just have to organise it around the house[6].'*

Disorganised approaches were typified by good intentions that never reached fruition, or reference to 'ad hoc' approaches at organisation:

> *'Well sometimes you say 'I'm going to do that tonight' then something comes along and you don't, and sometimes that's why I prefer something a bit structured, so that I'm not left to the end to get it all done. I like to think I'm on week one of month one or whatever[9].'*

> *'I just did it when I could, mainly Saturday afternoons or Sunday evenings[15].'*

> *'It was ad hoc, when I had time. I knew I couldn't put it off too long because my daughter typed it for me and my husband read it[16].'*

One student demonstrated a link between systematic wading and disorganised approaches to assignment management:

> *'I just plodded through* [the essay] *really and didn't analyse it. I'm not very good at structuring my work. I can't see the wood for the trees when I'm doing an assignment[11].'*

Disorganised approaches, therefore, seemed to be characterised by the need to be structured by an outside source, such as the learning materials themselves, official deadlines, or typing arrangements. The properties of the category of organisation are listed in *Table 4.6*.

Table 4.6: Properties associated with organisation

Category	Properties
Organised	Goal orientated (8) Use holidays for study (8)
Semi-organised	Organise study around shifts and family routine (7) Diverse study space includes work environment (7,6)
Disorganised	Use ad hoc approaches to study (15,16) Have good intentions that do not bear fruit (9) Need structure from external source (16)

The final part of the analysis was designed to ascertain what impact, if any, the characteristics already identified had on the level of learning achieved by students. Thus, the final concept 'level of learning' was generated.

Concept eleven—level of learning

Two levels of learning are evident in the literature—deep learning and surface learning (Marton and Saljo, 1976b), as discussed in *Chapter 2*. Marton and Saljo found that 'deep' and 'surface' approaches to learning emerged when students were asked to introspect about their experience of reading a text. Students' comments ranged from 'Well, I just concentrated on trying to remember as much as possible' (surface level) to '...I thought about how he had built up the whole thing' (deep level). In 'surface' level approaches, students focus on the 'sign'—a rote learning strategy; while in 'deep' level approaches, students are directed towards the intentional content of the material, i.e. what is signified (Marton and Saljo, 1976b). Saljo (1979a) concluded that, although most students consider both approaches to be relevant to their learning, depending on the context, some students are only capable of using a surface approach.

When asked what was meant by learning (Saljo, 1979a), students revealed five conceptions of learning—learning as increase in knowledge; memorising, acquiring facts, procedures, etc., to retain and use in practice; abstraction of meaning; and an interpretive process aimed at understanding reality. Qualitative differences between conceptions 2 and 3 and between 4 and 5 are similar to the distinction between surface and deep approaches (Gibbs *et al*,1982).

Marton and Saljo's (1976b) 'deep' and 'surface' levels of understanding also formed the basis of a phenomenological study (Morgan *et al*, 1982), which investigated approaches to study and implications for improving student learning of 29 Open University students. They interviewed respondents before, during, and after a foundation course. The 'deep' level approach was illustrated by a requirement for the reader to engage in a destructuring followed by restructuring of knowledge, so that the material is related to the student's own construct system. This approach corresponded to the fourth and fifth conceptions of learning (Saljo, 1979b), both of which involve active learning through 'abstraction of meaning' and 'interpretive processes aimed at understanding reality'.

The 'surface' level approaches included attempts to memorise material rather than engage with it. This confirms Marton and Saljo's (1979a) theory of 'horizontalisation', which focuses on *what* is attended to, so that students concentrate on all the text at the same level, in spite of the broad principles and specific details. This approach also supports Saljo's (1979a) theory of passive learning, which involves accumulation of information and memorising facts.

Most adult learners will have arrived at Saljo's third step, involving the distinction between learning and understanding, and this should facilitate the development of deeper-level approaches and, hence, more successful learning outcomes. Moreover, distance learners, who are studying while working in a profession, probably concur with the conceptions of learning (Saljo, 1979b) as increase in knowledge and acquiring facts, procedures, etc., to retain and use in practice. The deeper level approaches of abstraction of meaning, and an interpretive process aimed at understanding reality, are desirable conceptions that some students will probably achieve during degree level education.

In the study on which this book is based, a deep approach was characterised by the comment of one student when asked what she would do if she could not understand concepts:

> *'I'd try and look at it in a different way, in another book, get another book that's recommended reading and see another way of explaining it and then perhaps read it again[7].'*

This same student said that she remembered things by:

> *'Writing things down, I've always done it, it takes longer, but I find writing particular sentences and key words and writing and memorising, that's what I've always done at work as well as studying. It's as if it clarifies it in my head[7].'*

This comment could be categorised as both maximalist learning and systematic wading, while also demonstrating a link with deep learning. By contrast, surface learners were more passive in their use of the materials, as indicated by one student, who could also be defined as passive towards the learning process:

> *'The activities and things, I didn't do. I just basically read it, just as a source of literature really ... to look for the kind of topics that the subject covered and then just set about writing and answering the assignment question. So I didn't really have any intention of trying to remember what was in it. Basically at the end of the day it was a means to an end[1].'*

This student went on to say that she dislikes distance learning and learns better through exchange of ideas and group discussion, preferring both internal and external dialogue, and checklists to discuss with a tutor. The students' responses suggest that a desire to understand content could be the distinguishing feature between deep and surface learning, thus supporting the work of other authors (Saljo, 1979b; Morgan *et al*, 1982). This also indicates a link between depth of learning and view of knowledge. Students who view knowledge as sought by themselves, for example, seem more likely to engage in deep learning, than students who view knowledge as something that should be given to them.

The properties of the categories of deep and surface learning are listed in *Table 4.7*.

Table 4.7: Properties associated with deep and surface learning

Category	Properties
Deep learning	Attempt to deepen understanding during assignment completion (7) Taking time (7) Read widely to search for explanations (7)
Surface learning	Mainly concerned with completing the task (1) View knowledge as something that should be given to them (1) View learning as a means to an end (1) Dislike distance learning (1)

Results, this far, suggest that the way in which students approach their study in distance learning affects all other aspects of the learning process, from the need for guidance within and outside of materials, to the level of learning achieved. With such a complex array of concepts and categories, axial coding was then used to draw the findings together into a more coherent whole.

Summary

The qualitative analysis resulted in the development of concepts, categories and associated properties, which are presented in the tables above. Once this process was complete, axial coding (Strauss and Corbin, 1990) was used to draw links between the different categories and concepts. This enabled the data to be re-assembled in a way that might explain the needs for support and guidance for different types of students, and how this might affect the outcome of learning. 'The use of grounded theory demonstrates links between styles and strategies and how these are mediated by other concepts, such as the need for guidance and engagement with materials' (Carnwell, 2000a: 139).

Britt (1997) advises that it is important to decide which are the most important variables, what the nature of the variables and concepts are, and how they are related. This resulted in dividing the categories into three overarching concepts that reflected the most important links between concepts and categories. The three concepts are:

- need for guidance
- approaches to studying

- engagement with materials.

These three concepts produce a useful summary of the data.

Need for guidance

Students' need for guidance included characteristics that were shared with other concepts, such as preference for external dialogue, closed materials, an active tutor and the need for academic support. It was in the areas in which the same characteristics (or properties) were used to define different categories that links could be made.

External dialogue, while being linked to the need for guidance, was also linked with a desire for closed materials. Guidance, then, is necessary to help students to determine their learning needs and to find their way through the learning process. Furthermore, guidance can be by provided by either closed materials, or external dialogue. An important link is also observed between closed materials and self-help. This may indicate that closed materials provide sufficient guidance for some students, who would prefer to engage in self-help groups rather than have contact with a tutor.

The need for guidance was also linked to an active tutor role that was defined in relation to the tutor role, both within and outside of planned group tutorials. Within the planned group tutorial, the active tutor role involved the tutor actively teaching and controlling the direction of the tutorial. Outside of the tutorial, the active tutor role entailed the tutor being proactive in contacting students. A further defining attribute of the active tutor was the provision of specific assignment guidance either within or outside of the group tutorial. It may be concluded that some students will need high material structure, external dialogue, and for the tutor to take an active role. By comparison, other students require less material structure, less dialogue, and prefer academic support in the form of tutor availability and responsiveness, as long as adequate and appropriate information is provided.

A link was also found between external dialogue and commitment. Commitment was sub-divided into either maximalist or minimalist, both of which were linked to external dialogue, but for different reasons. Minimalist students needed to be disciplined by an external source. Maximalist students needed external dialogue as a source of feedback on aspects of their learning (e.g., writing style), rather than interaction.

A link existed between a preference for both types of dialogue and guidance throughout the learning process, as indicated by properties of fear and research jargon. These suggest that students lack confidence and have difficulty with materials, these being typical attributes of students needing both types of dialogue.

Approaches to studying

The three approaches to study were linked most closely with serialist and holist learning, since these had over-lapping properties.

Systematic waders tend to adopt a serialist approach to learning (Pask and Scott, 1972; see *Chapter* 2). Serialists and flexible serialists tend to be maximalist learners and, due to a desire to understand, will possibly read as instructed rather than prioritising their reading according to its relevance. Holists and flexible holists, like speedy-focussers and global dippers, tend to select their reading according to its relevance to the assignment or interest. However, they may change their natural approach to serialist learning if they perceive the materials as a 'programme of learning'. The structure of materials can, therefore, be important in enabling students to adopt a less preferred learning style.

By comparison, surface learners tend to use a minimalist approach to the materials; to prefer both types of dialogue; closed materials with checklists to discuss with a tutor; and to view knowledge as given. The characteristics of surface learning, then, seem to overlap with those of the global dipper.

The global dipper approach to study did appear to be the most problematic in terms of poor/adverse learning experiences. This should not imply that this approach to study itself is ineffective, since other factors, such as inexperience of study, or domestic circumstances could impact on students' natural approaches to study. A possible link could exist between global dipper approaches to study and organisation of study. Organised students were typically goal-orientated, whereas semi-organised approaches would be partly dictated by shift patterns and attempts to do some studying at work. Disorganised approaches were typified by good intentions that never reached fruition, or reference to 'ad hoc' approaches at organisation.

Engagement with materials

The concept 'engagement with materials' reflects the way in which students select their reading, the extent to which they actively engage in the reading they select, and the depth of learning that results from this process. Links can be seen between approaches to study and approaches to *learning* (i.e. level of learning achieved), relevance of reading, and engagement with materials. Systematic waders tend to use serialist approaches, to actively engage with materials, and to read as instructed. They are more likely to view knowledge as sought, and to engage in deep learning. Speedy-focussed learners are more likely to use holist or flexible holist approaches and will, therefore, select their reading according to its relevance to the essay. Global dippers will tend to be flexible serialists, will select their reading according to its relevance to the essay, and are more likely to be minimalist learners. Minimalist learning is associated with surface learning, the desire for closed materials, both types of dialogue, and a view of knowledge as 'given'.

These links reveal important distinctions relating to the three approaches to study in terms of type of guidance required, approaches to learning adopted, and engagement with materials. These links made it possible to delineate descriptions and attributes of the three approaches to study and how they impact on the need for guidance and engagement with materials (see *Table 4.8*).

Table 4.8: Descriptions and attributes of the three approaches to study

Approach to study	Description	Attributes relating to guidance and engagement with materials
Systematic wader	Reads systematically, taking few short cuts. 'Wades' through the materials and sometimes gets 'bogged down'. Is interested in content, enjoys learning and views knowledge as 'sought'	Closed materials combined with passive tutor role and academic support provide sufficient guidance Internal dialogue successful Serialist learning Read as instructed Active engagement with materials fosters deep learning

Approach to study	Description	Attributes relating to guidance and engagement with materials
Speedy-focusser	Focusses quickly on key points relevant to the assignment. Is a very efficient and effective learner. Is instrumental in learning and views knowledge as 'given'	Open materials and passive tutor role preferred. No dialogic preference Flexible holist approach to learning. Selects reading according to its relevance to the essay Only engages actively with certain parts of the materials, therefore engages in limited deep learning, as related to the essay
Global dipper	Begins systematically, but resorts to dipping in and out of the materials in search of clues to answer the question. Seeks advice from others, finds the learning process difficult. Views knowledge as 'given'	Need closed materials, both types of dialogue and an active tutor to provide necessary guidance Adopts flexible serialist approach to learning Selects reading according to the essay, but has difficulty making the selection Passively engages with the materials and anxiously seeks out a variety of external dialogue. Engages in surface learning

Having described the three approaches to study and identified their main attributes, the properties and dimensions of each approach to study were then listed in *Table 4.9*.

Table 4.9: Properties and dimensions of each approach to study

Approach to study	Property	Dimension
Systematic wader	Guidance Materials preference Dialogue Tutor role Reading selection Commitment Level of learning	Medium Closed Internal Passive No selection Maximalist Deep
Speedy-focusser	Guidance Materials preference Dialogue Tutor role Reading selection Commitment Level of learning	Low Open No preference Passive Relevance to essay Maximalist in parts Surface
Global-dipper	Guidance Materials preference Dialogue Tutor role Reading selection Engagement with material Level of learning	High Closed External and internal Active Relevance to essay Minimalist Surface

The analysis reveals some important distinctions between the three approaches to study. The three emerging concepts—guidance, approaches to study, and engagement with materials—proved useful in drawing these distinctions. It seems that the need for guidance differs between the three approaches to study. Moreover, guidance can be defined in relation to materials design, the role of the tutor and dialogic preferences, which provide a link between materials and tutor role. Students with different approaches to study approach their learning in distinctly different ways, and these approaches mediate between the need for guidance and engagement with the materials. Thus, students with different approaches to study might achieve differing levels of learning. A more detailed analysis and the development of predictive models of approaches to study, along with their implications for learning and teaching, can be found elsewhere (Carnwell, 2000b).

The next chapter will consider the implications of these findings for support for distance learners and the development of coping strategies in distance learning students. Before beginning *Chapter 5*, however, readers are invited to reflect on their own learning and how it affects their needs for support and guidance in the following activities.

Reflection

Think about the way in which you normally approach your learning, then consider which of the three approaches to study most closely resembles your own.

How does your approach to study affect other aspects of your learning, including:

- The type of guidance you require within learning materials, from your tutor, and from peers
- Your need for support and from where you acquire it
- The way in which you organise your study
- The level of learning you feel you normally achieve.

Practical activity

In the light of the above reflection, draw up an action plan to include the following:

- How you intend to use distance learning materials, given your preferences for structure of materials
- How you intend to negotiate with your tutor to ensure that your learning needs are met, both within and outside of tutorials
- How you intend to access appropriate support, and from whom you will acquire this
- Your plans to keep the progress of your study on course.

References

Bailey D (1992) Facilitator not teacher: A role for tutors in open learning nurse education. *J Adv Nurs* **17**: 983–91

Bailey D, Moore J (1989) Closing the distance: Counselling at O.U. residential schools. *J Guid Counsel* **17**(3): 317–30

Bernard RM, Lundgren KM (1994) Learner assessment and text design strategies for distance education. *Can J Educat Comm* **23**(2): 133–52

Britt DW (1997) *A Conceptual Introduction to Modelling: Qualitative and Quantitative Perspectives.* Lawrence Erlbraum Associates, Publishers, Mahwah, NJ

Burge L (1988) Beyond androgogy: Some explorations for distance learning design. *J Dist Educ* **3**(1): 5–23

Canfield A, Lafferty J (1974) *Learning Style Inventory.* M I Experimental Learning Methods, Plymouth

Carnwell R (2000a) Approaches to study and their impact on the need for support and guidance in distance learning. *Open Learn* **15**(2): 123–40

Carnwell R (2000b) Pedagogical implications of approaches to study in distance learning: Developing models through qualitative and quantitative analysis. *J Adv Nurs* **31**(5): 1018–28

Evans T, Nation D (1989) Dialogue in practice, research and theory in distance education. *Open Learn* **4**(2): 37–42

Garrison DR, Baynton M (1987) Beyond independence in distance education: The concept of control. *Am J Dist Educ* **1**(3): 3–15

Gibbs G, Lockwood F, Morgan A, Taylor E (1982) Student learning and course design 1: In-text devices in Open University texts. *Study Methods Group Report*, No. 12. Institute of Educational Technology, Open University, Milton Keynes

Hargreaves D (1978) The significance of classroom coping strategies. In: Barton L, Meighan R, eds. *Socialogical Interpretations of Schooling and Classroom: A Reapraisal*. Nafferton Books, Driffield: 73–100

Harrison B, Jr (1997) Hardware/software to support distance learning classes 6 p., In: *Mid-South Instructional Technology Conference Proceedings* (2nd, Murfreesboro, TN, April 6-8, (1997); see IR 019 485; http://www.mtsu.edu/~itconf/proceed97/harrison.html

Hartley J (1988a) Using principles of text design to improve the effectiveness of audiotapes. *Br J Educat Technol* **19**(1): 4–16

Hartley J (1988b) *Designing Instructional Text* (2nd edn). Kogan Page and Nichols Publishing, London

Holmberg B (1989) *Theory and Practice of Distance Education*. Routledge, London

Johnson, William T (1999) Library Support for Distance Learning. Community & Junior College Libraries. v8 n2 p51–7

Kelly P (1987) Tutorial groups in open learning. In: Thorpe M, Grugeon D, (eds). *Open Learning For Adults*. Longman, Harlow/Essex: 275–92

Kirkup G, von Prummer C (1990) Support and connectedness: The needs of women distance education students. *J Dist Educ* **5**(2): 9–31

Kommers PAM, Lenting BF, van der Veer GG (1998) Distributed collaborative learning in a Telematic context. Telematic learning support and its potential for collaborative learning with new paradigms and conceptual mapping tools. *Educat Media Int* **35**(3): 100–5

Lebel C (1989) Le support a l'etudiant en enseignement a distance. *J Dist Educ* **IV**(2): 7–24

Leornard A, Jowett J (1990) *Project 2000–1, Charting the Course: A Study of 6 ENB Pilot Schemes in Pre-Registration Nurse Education*. National Foundation for Educational Research in England and Wales, Slough

Martens R *et al* (1996) Functions, use and effects of embedded support devices. *Learn Instr* **6**(1): 77–93

Marton F, Saljo R (1976a) On qualitative differences in learning I: Outcome and process. *Br J Educat Psychol* **46**: 4–11

Marton F, Saljo R (1976b) On qualitative differences in learning II: Outcome as a function of the learner's perception of the task. *Br J Educat Psychol* **46**: 115–27

Merritt SL (1983) Learning style preferences of Baccalaureate nursing students. *Nurs Res* **32**(6): 367–72

Moore MG (1973) Toward a theory of independent learning and teaching. *J High Educ* **XLIV**(12): 661–79

Moore M (1990) Recent contributions to the theory of distance education. *Open Learn* **5**(3): 10–15

Morgan A, Taylor E, Gibbs G (1982) Variations in students' approaches to studying. *Br J Educ Technol* **2**(13): 107–13

Pascoe EJ (1977) *For Older College Women*. McCall Publishing Co, LA, California

Pask G, Scott BCE (1972) Learning strategies and individual competence. *Int J Man-Mach Stud* **4**: 212–53

Payton OD, Hueter AE, Mcdonald ME (1979) Learning style preferences of physical therapy students in the United States. *Physic Ther* **59**: 147–52

Perraton H (1985) A theory of distance education. In: Sewart D, Keegan D, Holmberg B (eds). *Distance Education: International Perspectives.* Croom Helm, Beckenham, Kent: 34–45

Pym FR (1992) Women and distance education: A nursing perspective. *J Adv Nurs* **17**: 383–9

Pym FR, Atkinson AM (1990) Reaching out via distance education to nurses: Needs assessment, planning and implications. Paper presented at the Third Congress of the Canadian Association for Distance Education, Quebec City. In: Pym FR (1992) Women and distance education: A nursing perspective. *J Adv Nurs* **17**: 383–89

Riechmann SW, Grasha AF (1974) A rational approach to developing and assessing the construct validity of a student learning styles scale instrument. *J Psychol* **87**: 213–23

Sadler-Smith E (1997) Learning style: Frameworks and instruments. *Educat Psychol* **17**(1&2): 51–63

Saljo R (1979a) Learning in the learner's perspective: IV Considering one's own strategy. Report from the Institute of Education. University of Goteborg, No. 79. In: Gibbs G, Morgan A, Taylor E (1982) A review of the research of Ference Marton and the Goteborg group: A phenomenological research perspective on learning. *High Educ* **11**: 123–45

Saljo R (1979b) Learning in the learner's perspective: II Differences in awareness. Reports from the Institute of Education. University of Goteborg, No. 77. In: Gibbs G, Morgan A, Taylor E (1982) A review of the research of Ference Marton and the Goteborg group: A phenomenological research perspective on learning. *High Educat* **11**: 123–45

Sewart D (1987) Limitations of the learning package. In: Thorpe M, Grugeon D (eds). *Open Learning for Adults.* Longman, Harlow, Essex: 31–7

Simpson O (1993) Quality in distance learning support—some questions, a few points, no answers. *Open Learn* **8**(2): 61–3 (June)

Strauss A, Corbin J (1990) *Basics of Qualitative Research: Grounded Theory Procedures and Techniques.* Sage, London

Vowles B (1990) Educational guidance. *Conference Proceedings of Student Learning in the Open University—Process and Practice.* Open University Press, Milton Keynes

5
Coping strategies of women distance learners

Introduction

Chapter 4 discussed how students with different approaches to study had differing needs for guidance and support. Moreover, accessing the appropriate support mechanisms is important in helping students to gain maximum benefit from learning materials so that they can achieve a higher level outcome. It is proposed here, that women distance learners not only access the support they need, but also develop coping strategies to help them to move through the learning process successfully. This chapter will first examine some of the literature pertaining to supporting students in distance learning, and will then explore the coping strategies used by women distance learners.

Section one—supporting students in distance learning

In *Chapter 4,* three different types of support emerged from the interviews—practical support, emotional support, and academic support. Support appeared to be important to the students studied and this is confirmed by other studies discussed in *Chapter 1* (Pym, 1992; Pym and Atkinson, 1990; Kirkup and von Prummer, 1990). Although women students view support as important, their performance is equal to or better than that of younger students. In fact, Pascoe (1977) quotes one interview respondent, a professor, as stating that the mature woman 'works harder, digs deeper and gets more out of college than any other group of students' (p45), while another respondent said, 'they're earnest, they study harder, they contribute more, their papers are better'. For women working full-time while studying, work patterns can make it even more difficult to find blocks of time to study, and this factor makes the need for support in distance learning an important part of the learning process.

The three types of support identified in this research, together with the above evidence, indicate the need to explore the concept of support further, and to attempt to *measure* support needs of women distance learners. Support tends to be defined in terms of its constituents (Carnwell *et al*, 2001). Carnwell *et al* categorise the literature concerning definitions of support in terms of *activities* (Bailey and Moore, 1989), *strategies* (Lebel, 1989), and *skills* (Vowles, 1990) that enable students to progress satisfactorily. *Activities* might include seeking support from various sources, *strategies* can be divided into cognitive, affective, metacognitive and motivational and *skills* include informing, advising, counselling, assessing, enabling, and feeding back.

The attempts to *measure* support needs led to the development of a Learning Support Needs Questionnaire (LSNQ) (Moreland and Carnwell, 2000; Carnwell *et al*, 2001). The LSNQ draws on all three of the above constituents—activities, strategies and skills. Answers to items in part one of the instrument provide tutors with information that will assist them to advise, counsel, and assess students more accurately. Part two of the LSNQ involves an action plan, which students complete to identify activities and strategies that enable them to progress successfully. The LSNQ, therefore, does not only *measure* support needs, but also, through use of the action plan, helps students to *connect* with different support services. The need for students to *connect* with tutors and course writers arose from their expressed preferences for dialogue, both internal to the packages (i.e. through in-text activities) and external to the package (i.e. with other students and tutors) (Carnwell, 1999). The concept of *connectedness* has also been explored in other studies (Lawton, 1997; Stark and Warne, 1999).

Lawton develops a theoretical model of supportive learning in which connectedness is achieved through regular personal contact between student and tutor. Lawton identifies four variables within this relationship, as follows:

- the student variable, which involves self-confidence and independent learning skills

- the student-student variable, which involves networking with other students and tutors
- the tutor variable, in which tutors should be knowledgeable, adaptable, available, and credible
- the course content variable, which includes provision of pre-course information and joint planning of individual programmes of study.

Within this model, the student and tutor move through three phases of their relationship—the meeting phase, the guiding phase, and, finally, the 'moving on' phase (Lawton, 1997). These three phases mirror the phases of a model proposed by Peplau (1952). During the meeting phase, learning needs are assessed and expectations discussed. The second phase, which appeared to be important to the students discussed in *Chapter 4,* is characterised by tutors marking and returning work and providing feedback on progress. Lawton comments on the need for a trusting relationships, so that students do not feel as though they are being a burden or 'bothering' the tutor—a concern that was expressed by one of the participants cited in *Chapter 4*. The final phase involves the parting of students and tutors, while acknowledging the learning that has taken place. It is through this combination of interactions, within the context of the course, that connectedness takes place and support is experienced.

Distance learning, however, can, by its very nature, limit the amount of connectedness that can take place, as indicated in a study by Stark and Warne (1999). In Stark and Warne's study of 70 students (mainly mature nurses), opportunities to 'connect' with university tutors were limited to face-to-face tutorials, telephone calls, and submission of written work assessment. Data from focus-group interviews and conversations with students revealed that they felt 'disconnected' from the institution, and that this led them to divert their energies towards family commitments. They expected tutors to be interested in them as individuals and to provide reassurance, support, advice, and motivation. Interviews of tutors revealed that they, too, found that some students felt 'disconnected' from the university, and this affected the quality of their assignments. Tutors commented that students needed to know what they (the tutors) would be looking for in their assignments. Students also needed contact numbers to provide reassurance, supportive handouts to take away, and an opportunity to network and 'connect' with other students who had similar feelings (Stark and Warne, 1999). These findings mirror comments of students in *Chapter 4* in their preference for tutor roles, such as an active tutor or self-help groups. In Stark and Warne's research, tutors also commented that the apparent 'disconnectedness' in some students might have been due to the emphasis on course content rather than the student, which, they argue, dehumanised the learning experience and created dependence. The concept of 'connectedness' was viewed as crucial to distance learning (Stark and Warne, 1999). This was sub-divided into three themes, the first two of which resemble the first two phases outlined by Lawton (1997):

- continuity, in which the same tutor meets with the same group of students at each study day (this resembles Lawton's meetings phase)
- structure, in which university regulations, dates and deadlines are made explicit (this resembles Lawton's guiding phase)
- a 'human touch', which includes genuineness, caring and commitment to students.

The evidence suggests that support is important to women distance learners in enabling them to *connect* with other people who will facilitate their progress. It would appear that achieving this 'connectedness' is the responsibility of both the student and the institution. Students bear the responsibility for diagnosing their own needs for support and making contact with support services, and the institution is responsible for making high quality support services and guidance available. It is further argued above, that support needs can be measured, so that students can be more self-aware of their needs and so that tutors can respond more appropriately to students with different types of support need. Support, however, exists within a context, and for women distance learners, the context is usually that of domestic responsibility. As Pym

(1992) points out, women carry the main burden of domestic responsibility whether they are employed or not. Indeed, homemaking demands are not reduced when a woman engages in study (Green, 1987). It is proposed, therefore, that despite attempts to diagnose student support needs and to provide support services to meet them, women will also develop coping strategies to enable them to cope with the demands of distance learning study.

Section two—coping strategies used by women distance learners

Before considering the coping strategies used by the distance learners in this study, it is first necessary to explore what 'coping' means.

Definitions and theories of coping

Cohen and Lazarus (1979: 219) define coping as, 'efforts, both action-oriented and intra-psychic, to manage (that is, master, tolerate, reduce and minimise) environmental and internal demands, and conflicts among them, which tax or exceed a person's resources'. A simpler definition of coping, is offered by Pearlin and Schooler (1978) as the 'things that people do to avoid being harmed by life strains' (p2). When learning at a distance, it is assumed that students do certain things to reduce the demands placed upon them, and to resolve conflicts arising from the competing demands of study and family life. Key to Cohen and Lazarus's (1979) definition, is that the coping strategies students use tend to come into play when demands exceed their resources to deal with them. The nature of this transaction between demands, and resources to meet them, makes coping strategies appealing to study for both psychologists and sociologists.

In psychological literature, coping strategies are closely allied to theories of stress and are viewed in this context as helping individuals to adapt during periods of stress (Holahan and Moos, 1987). From a sociological perspective, Pearlin and Schooler (1978) argue that understanding coping enables us to understand the impact that societies exert on their members. For Pearlin and Schooler, social roles cause life strains and people respond to these strains by adopting coping modes that are shared by people with key social characteristics.

These two competing approaches to the understanding of coping are reflected in the various attempts to measure coping. Typically, psychological literature consists of different scales to measure coping. An example of this is Carver *et al*'s (1989) theoretically based instrument (COPE). Having identified questionnaire items from psychological literature, Carver *et al* distributed the final set of items to 978 undergraduates at the University of Miami. The results were then subjected to factor analysis, which resulted in questionnaire items being divided into different sections—active coping, planning, suppression of competing alternatives, restraint coping, seeking social support, focussing on and venting emotions, and behavioural disengagement. An interesting finding was that the more the situation mattered to subjects, the more likely they were to vent emotions, engage in denial, and seek out social support.

Carver *et al*'s COPE inventory was later adapted by Adejumo and Brysiewicz (1998) for the purpose of studying coping strategies of Baccalaureate nursing students. They argued that knowledge of methods used by students to cope with stressful situations would enable educators to guide them and provide them with, either their usual comfortable strategies, or alternative workable strategies. Adejumo and Brysiewicz's study was, thus, based on Carver *et al*'s assertion that people cope better when they are able to turn to familiar and comfortable strategies, rather than when these strategies are not available. Their adaptation of the COPE inventory (Carver *et al*, 1989) resulted in items deemed to measure problem-focussed coping (see *Table 5.1*), emotion-focussed coping (see *Table 5.2*); and dysfunctional (not-very-useful) coping strategies (see *Table 5.3*). Adejumo and Brysiewicz's three categories are similar to the three categories identified by Holahan and Moos (1987). Holahan and Moos compared depressed patients (n=395) with matched controls of comparable socio-economic status (405) using a questionnaire survey. The three types of coping strategy they identified were *active-cognitive strategies, active-behavioural strategies*, and *avoidance strategies*.

Table 5.1: Items measuring problem-focussed coping

Item	Example
Active coping	Deliberate increase in effort to achieve a goal
Planning	Pausing to consider how to deal with a problematic situation
Suppression of competing activities	Deliberately putting aside other things in order to focus on the stressor related to academic work
Restraint coping	Forcing one to wait until the right time, rather than acting immediately
Seeking of social support	Asking others how to solve a problem relating to an assignment

Adejumo and Brysiewicz's (1998) *problem-focussed* strategies are similar to Holahan and Moos's (1987) *active-behavioural strategies*. These include:

- trying to find out more about the situation
- talking with someone about the problem
- busying self with other things to take mind off the problem
- getting away from things for a while.

Both problem-focussed and active-behavioural strategies are active in nature and rely on doing things, such as making contact with other people, or changing one's own activities.

Table 5.2: Items measuring emotion-focussed coping

Item	Example
Seeking emotional support	Seeking moral support, sympathy or understanding, not what to do
Positive re-interpretation	Desire to see positive side of what is happening, so that individual can be spurred on to achieve desired goal
Acceptance	By accepting the situation the person is more likely to deal with it or accommodate to it
Denial	Refusal to believe the existence of a real stressor
Turning to religion	Turning to God, or other supernatural beings during stress

Adejumo and Brysiewicz's (1998) *emotion-focussed* strategies are similar to Holahan and Moos's (1987) *active-cognitive strategies*. These strategies include:

- praying for guidance
- preparing for the worst
- considering alternative ways of handling the problem
- drawing on past experience.

Both of these strategies rely on thinking about the problem in order to find a solution.

Table 5.3: Items measuring dysfunctional strategies

Item	Example
Focus on, and venting of, emotions	Talking about one's feelings and focussing on distress
Behavioural disengagement	Giving up activities that will lead to achievement of goals
Mental disengagement	Day-dreaming, sleep, immersion in activities that will distract from problems
Alcohol-drug disengagement	Escape through alcohol or drugs to take mind off the problem

Adejumo and Brysiewicz's (1998) *dysfunctional* strategies are similar to Holahan and Moos's (1987) *avoidance strategies*, which include:

- taking it out on other people
- avoiding being with people
- drinking or eating more to reduce tension.

Again these categories are very similar, with a reliance on venting of emotions, disengagement and alcohol. It is particularly interesting that the three categories of these studies bear so much similarity given the different groups studied (i.e. Baccalaureate nursing students and depressed patients).

The findings of Adejumo and Brysiewicz's study revealed that the top three strategies used by students were planning, turning to religion and seeking social support. Furthermore, a mixture of coping strategies that combined problem-focussed and emotion-focussed strategies was often used. Within the dysfunctional category, venting of emotions was most commonly used. The authors acknowledge Carver *et al*'s argument that this can be effective in facilitating adaptation to the situation, while recognising that prolonged focussing can impede emotional adjustment, as argued by Scheier and Carver (1977). Abouserie (1996) also found similar evidence when she measured coping strategies in relation to job satisfaction of academic staff (n= 414). She found that academic staff use a range of coping strategies to deal with stress and often several strategies are used simultaneously, or in sequence, to support each other. Some strategies seemed to be focussed towards reducing the emotional discomfort associated with stress, rather than reducing its cause. The highest scoring strategies were: acceptance of the problem (58%), talking with others (57.7%), trying to come to terms with each problem (55.8%), involving self with friends (51.7%), trying to say no to unnecessary demands (51.7%), and talking about it with colleagues (43.5%).

The findings of Holahan and Moos's (1987) study revealed that active coping strategies (both cognitive and behavioural) are associated with more personal and contextual resources (e.g. self-confidence and family support), whereas avoidance coping strategies are associated with fewer resources. They also found that easy-going individuals are less likely to rely on avoidance coping strategies.

Each of these studies, although using psychological dimensions and scales, reveals the significance of social support as a coping mechanism. This seems to confirm the importance of sociological studies that attempt to consider the situation, as well as the individual. A study that addresses this issue was conducted by Pearlin and Schooler (1978), who interviewed 2300 people in Chicago between ages 18–65 years about how they cope with ordinary adverse social experiences. From these interviews they identified three major types of coping:

- Responses that change the situation out of which strainful experience arises
- Responses that control the meaning of the strainful experience after it occurs, but before the emergence of stress

- Responses that function more for the control of stress itself after it has emerged (p9).

The authors argue that responses, which modify the situation (the first category) are most successful, as they attempt to eliminate the source of the stress. When it is not possible to alter the source of the stress, the second category aims to control the meaning of the problem, such as gaining solace from comparing self with others who feel the same way. This seemed to be a coping strategy of students who used a global dipper approach to study, and who often referred to the fact that other students felt the same way. This type of coping functions merely to help people accommodate to existing stress without being overwhelmed by it. It will not alter the situation, or the perceptions of it, and includes strategies, such as acceptance of the situation, and avoiding confrontation. An interesting finding in Pearlin and Schooler's (1978) study, is that coping was found to be least effective in areas of life, such as job, in which the stressful forces were beyond the control of the individual. The authors also distinguished between the *psychological resources* people use and things they *do* to cope with stress. They found that psychological resources are more important when dealing with things over which they have little control, such as job, whereas when dealing with situations in which they have more control, such as close interpersonal relationships, it is the things one does that make the difference. This might be why women distance learners often find it easier to divert energy away from study (requiring psychological resources) and towards practical tasks within the home, which will ease stress within family life.

The various studies reveal the importance of coping strategies in enabling people to manage stressful situations, such as study. There are a variety of instruments to measure coping strategies. Indeed, Cohen (1987) lists no less than fourteen such instruments. Despite these attempts to measure coping, however, Cohen concludes that there is insufficient correlation between similar instruments and insufficient evidence of validity to suggest the best measurements. Cohen further argues that there is insufficient evidence showing which coping dimensions are important to include within a scale. Some checklists, for example, are criticised for including too many items, and others for including too few. This book cannot propose the use of a particular measure of coping. The findings of the various studies do, however, allow some understanding of how and why women adopt certain coping strategies when combining study with full-time work.

In the light of the findings of various studies discussed above, it would seem that students navigate their way through the learning process using coping strategies, and that these are mediated by individual characteristics (e.g. approaches to study) and situational variables (e.g. home and work circumstances). Moreover, for women distance learners working full-time at the same time as engaging in part-time study, the impact of social circumstances may be an important influence on the coping strategies adopted. This social context influences the ability of the student to integrate the demands of part-time study into commitments of work, family and social life (Kember, 1995). Context, then, is likely to support the development of certain coping strategies resulting in a range of consequences, such as successful/unsuccessful learning experience, or enjoyable/unenjoyable learning experiences. The concept of coping strategy for this book is defined as things that students do to reduce the demands placed upon them, and to resolve conflicts arising from the competing demands of study and family life.

An alternative view of coping strategies, which takes account of social context, is that of Hargreaves' (1978: 77) who argues that:

> *'The essence of a model organised around the concept of coping strategy is that all actors... act meaningfully and creatively in response to their experienced world'.*

This holds true for the research on which this book is based, in that the different approaches to study and associated coping strategies reflect the way in which students respond creatively to their varied experiences. Using this model of coping strategies, it is proposed that the challenge of distance learning creates 'problems' for women distance learners. This causes them to devise a set of learning tactics and methods that will make life bearable (i.e. enable them to cope during the period of study) and outcomes achievable.

Furthermore, approaches to study will be generated and sustained only in so far as they enable successful coping with 'experienced constraints' (p77). Solutions that work will become taken-for-granted as a definition of learning. Solutions that do not work will be abandoned in favour of alternative solutions (Knowles, 1980). Hargreaves developed a 'coping cycle' (see *Figure 5.1*), which reflected the impact of context on coping strategies. Although Hargreaves' coping cycle was initially used to explain coping strategies used by teachers, it does have salience for distance learning.

As *Figure 5.1* suggests, teachers have to cope with a variety of institutional constraints arising from education and social structure, which are mediated by a range of variables such as age, level and social class. Like the teachers in Hargreaves' example, adult distance learners also have to cope with a variety of constraints. Hargreaves (1978) identifies constraints, such as contradictory goals within the educational system (p78), material constraints (p82), and a proliferation of educational ideologies to which teachers must respond (p87) as the major constraints faced by teachers. These constraints mirror those faced by women distance learners who are also working full-time. Contradictory goals emerge at an institutional level, between the need to gain higher educational qualifications, while continuing to work full-time, most often without study time being allowed. Like Hargreaves' example, these contradictory goals are managed by guided discovery, in this case through distance learning.

The material constraints faced by women distance learners concerns the lack of resources at both an institutional and personal level. As indicated in *Chapter 4*, at the institutional level, support mechanisms, in terms of academic support, are not always as available as students would like them to be. At an individual level, time and space, together with the demands of domestic and working life, are the main material constraints. Although distance learning provides flexibility to manage personal constraints, students have to develop coping

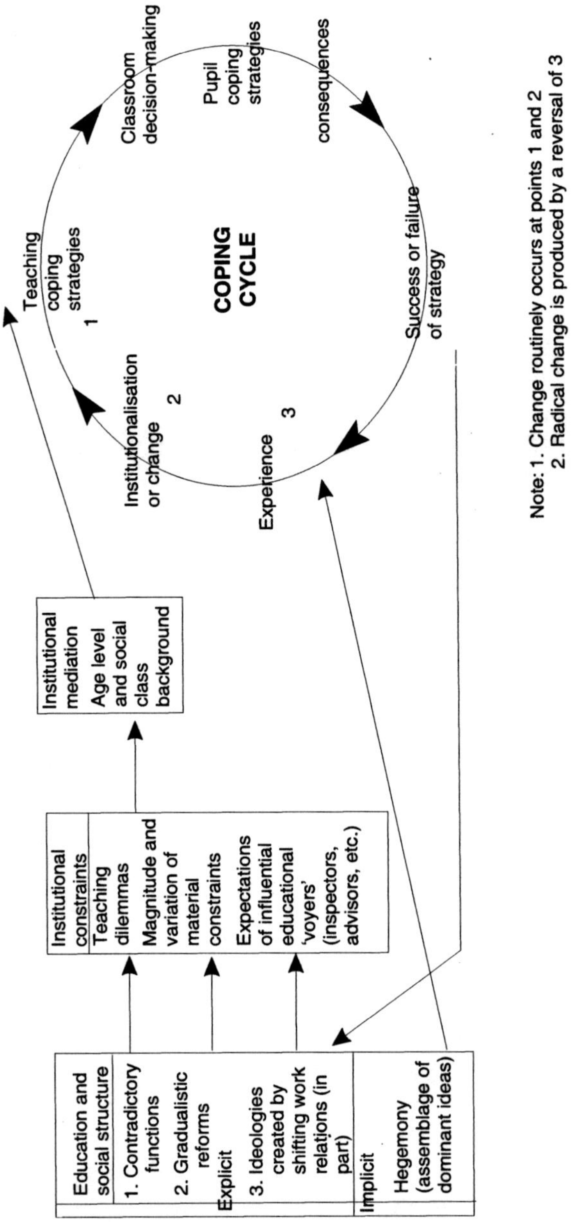

Figure 5.1: Hargreaves (1978) coping cycle(reproduced with the kind permission of Nafferton Books, Driffield)

strategies to manage their learning activities within the time allotted at the end of the working day, and within the constraints of domestic and family life. Such constraints are reflected in the importance of the need for practical support, which frequently arose as important in the interview data. Finally, the changing ideologies faced by this particular sample of women distance learners arose from changes in nurse education, in which first level nurses are now educated at diploma level, and community nurses at degree level. This change resulted in an educational momentum that created aspirations for most community nurses to acquire degree level status. For many nurses this involves distance learning study.

Hargreaves (1978) argues that these constraints are institutionally mediated. Like the children in Hargreaves' study, who were frequently called away to do something unrelated to their current task, women distance learners are frequently called away from their studies to attend to domestic chores, requests of family members, or work commitments. Tensions arising from women's role in domestic life are, therefore, both within the family and between the family and working life. Furthermore, although coping mechanisms are constructive and creative in character, they are also based on a set of tacitly accepted taken-for-granted assumptions about schooling, children, and learning—they are constructed within parameters such that the scope of creativity is limited (Hargreaves, 1978:94). Taken-for-granted assumptions include the perception that schooling and learning are, predominantly, for children. Although these boundaries have been challenged by trends in adult education, the philosophy of distance learning, with its home-based orientation, appears not to challenge, sufficiently, the parameters surrounding learning, work, and family life. It appears, therefore, that adult distance learners have to creatively construct coping strategies to re-define or to work within these parameters of constraints.

Hargreaves' model was adapted as a model to explain the coping cycle used by adult students undertaking distance learning programmes (see *Figure 5.2*).

The coping cycle, used for this study, also includes an inner circle that is divided into four quadrants reflecting the

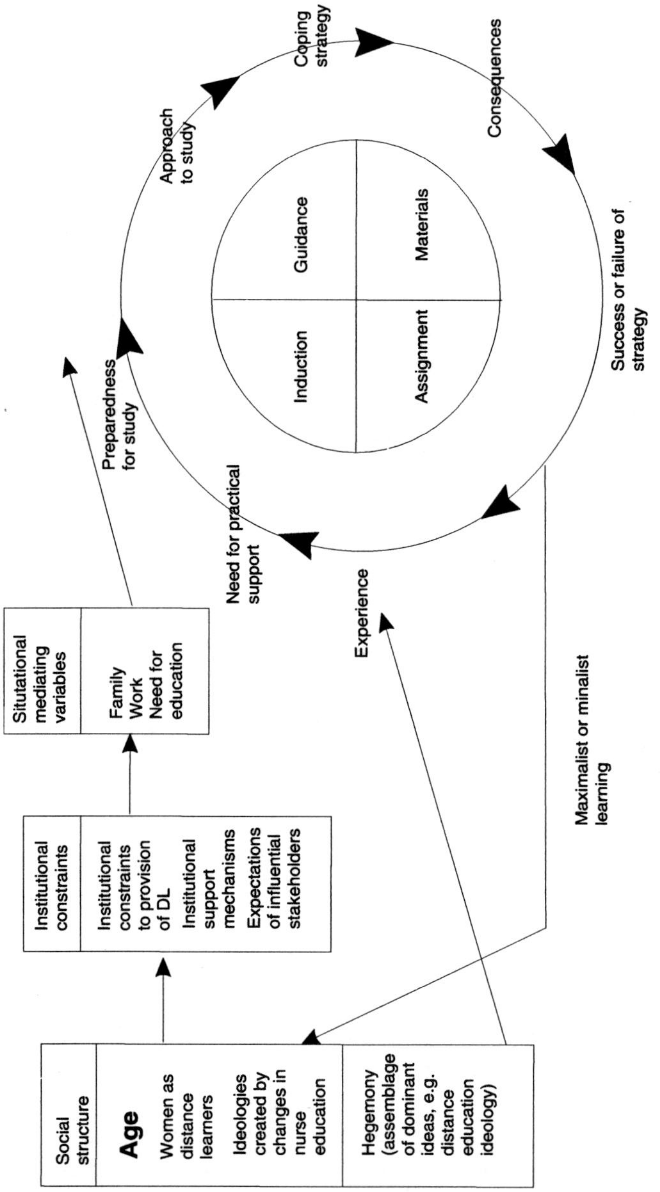

Figure 5.2: Coping cycle used by adult distance learners—adapted from Hargreaves (1978)

distance learning context: induction, guidance, materials-design and assignment preparation. The 'induction' quadrant reflects the need for students to be sufficiently prepared for study, which could enhance their coping strategies during the early part of the coping cycle. The 'guidance' quadrant responds to students' needs for dialogue (internal or external), which will also facilitate their coping, if provided in the appropriate form. Some students require guidance provided by internal dialogue and a passive tutor, and/or access to self-help groups. Others need guidance provided by active tutorial support and external dialogue. Diagnosing the nature of guidance needed during the preparation stage would begin the process that would be continued during the second stage. This would correspond to the student's particular approach to study, which is adjacent to guidance on the outer circle of the coping cycle.

Guidance is closely related to materials design (the third quadrant), since the materials can either help or hinder students in their study strategies, depending on their approach to learning. This corresponds to a stage in the outer circle of the model when students' coping strategies (mediated by the inner quadrants of the model, as well as external social, institutional, and situational constraints) have consequences that result in them either continuing or changing their study strategies. In turn, this leads to different approaches to assignment completion (the final inner quadrant), the consequence of which will be either a favourable or unfavourable learning experience. Coping strategies might include: an assignment focus in the reading of materials, a tendency to read as instructed, a deep or surface approach to understanding, a maximalist or minimalist approach to reading, and an organised or disorganised approach to assignment completion.

According to the model (*Figure 5.2*, adaptation is never complete and the 'cycle of coping' is never closed and static. Under these conditions, the cycle itself 'contains an internal dynamic and, like a bicycle wheel, advances as it rotates' (Hargreaves, 1978: 94). The 'external' dynamic of the model can be described as social, structural factors, institutional constraints, and situational variables that provide the context and parameters for individual action. According to Hargreaves, change will occur if coping strategies prove inefficient, in which case new ones will be devised. This allows for some variation in the degree of adaptation, but leaves the principle of adaptation intact. It is this principle of adaptation that is crucial in moving coping strategies beyond psychological measurement, and towards consideration of the interaction between the individual and the context in which learning takes place.

The literature on coping strategies has demonstrated its significance in moving beyond support mechanisms in distance learning. Furthermore, the limitation of psychological theories of coping has been emphasised. In distance learning settings, coping strategies based on socio-structural theories appear to be most useful. The next section will use three case studies to attempt to apply the theories discussed above.

Section three—demonstrating coping strategies using case studies

Three case studies (using pseudonyms), taken from the interviews discussed in *Chapters* 3 and 4, demonstrate application of the different theories of coping to distance learning. This demonstrates how students, with different approaches to study, use different coping strategies to adapt to the situation in which they find themselves.

Anna's case study explains relationships in Hargreaves' (1978) coping strategy model. She responded to the expectations of stakeholders in trying to advance her career prospects through distance learning, which she has since achieved. She has a family and work commitments and has a need for practical support at home. These factors provide the situational variables and context for her approach to study. She prepared herself for study, needed minimal guidance, and was satisfied with open materials. As a systematic wader, she used a serialist approach to learning, was rigorous, and demonstrated maximalist commitment to the materials. This 'coping strategy' was successful and enabled her to progress to further study. By engaging in further study, she contributed to the prevailing ideology in nurse education that graduate education is necessary, thus perpetuating the cycle in which social structures, institutional constraints, and situational variables impact on coping strategies. Anna's method of coping could be described as problem-focussed (Adejumo and Brysiewicz, 1998) in that she increased her efforts to achieve her goal, by systematically wading through the materials.

Bev's case study also validates Hargreaves' (1978) coping cycle model. She responded to institutional pressure to gain the required credits as access to a community health degree. Lack of institutional support acted as a constraint, as she was working full-time throughout her study. However, her situational context of having no family probably resulted in her needing little or no practical support and may also have contributed to her being well-organised. Her good organisation, combined with preparation for study, probably reduced her need for guidance. She adopted a speedy-focussed approach to study that allowed her to traverse the coping cycle efficiently and effectively. The consequence of this coping strategy was successful, in that it enabled her to pass the course, although she did not enjoy the learning experience, and, to a large extent, engaged in surface learning. Bev's coping strategy, therefore, bears some resemblance to Pearlin and Schooler's (1978: 9) three types of coping. The speedy-focussed approach could be used to 'change the situation out of which strainful experience arises', i.e., by adapting the nature of the learning package to meet her need to work quickly, she prevented the strain of study becoming uncomfortable and eliminated the source of stress. The fact that she did not enjoy the learning experience, however, might suggest that she did not modify the learning situation quickly enough. This might suggest use of Pearlin and Schooler's (1978: 9) second category in adopting a response to 'control the meaning of the strainful experience after it occurs, but before the emergence of stress'. For Bev, a more successful coping strategy might have been to adopt Adejumo and Brysiewicz's (1998) problem-focussed strategies. Active coping, for example, would have involved increased effort to achieve her goal, while planning would have enabled her to pause to consider how to deal with her learning. The seeking of social support would include asking others, such as students and tutors, how to solve a problem relating to an assignment. The combination of these three strategies might have resulted in a higher level of commitment to the materials.

Hargreaves' (1978) coping cycle can also be confirmed by Kay's case. She was pressurised to embark on the course by institutional policy, which actively encouraged/required community nurses of her grade to achieve diploma status. She had work commitments, needed practical support, and was not adequately prepared for study. These institutional constraints and situational variables provide the context for her experience. Her need for guidance and closed materials was high and was confirmed by her global dipper approach to study, which led her to use a strategy of flexible serialist learning to read the materials. The consequence of this, initially, was unsuccessful. Consequently, Kay changed her strategy to holist learning and then, later, to searching for clues from a variety of sources when this, too, proved unsuccessful. Although this strategy is an active-cognitive strategy (Holahan and Moos, 1987), in that it involves considering alternative ways of handling the problem, it is also typical of the dysfunctional strategy (Adejumo and Brysiewicz, 1998) of disengaging by giving up on activities that would lead to achievement of goals. Examples of this disengagement include giving up reading learning materials, in favour of other sources of information that often proved to be less relevant. Kay's coping strategies also included emotion-focussed coping (Adejumo and Brysiewicz, 1998), such as seeking moral support, sympathy or understanding, and the dysfunctional strategy of venting emotions. The use of these strategies resulted in Kay progressing around Hargreaves' cycle a number of times, before she adopted a strategy that enabled her to conclude her studies.

The three case studies reveal the importance of the different approaches to study in determining the different coping strategies used by students. The case studies also demonstrate the value of the different theories of coping strategies in relation to distance learning.

Summary

The particular difficulties of women distance learners have been well-documented. These include: balancing study with domestic chores and paid employment, isolation, and lack of support. Previous chapters have identified needs for support to assist students to cope with the competing demands placed upon them. This chapter concludes that students do not only gain access to support, but also develop coping strategies to help them to progress through the learning process. Both psychologists and sociologists have studied coping strategies. This chapter attempts to unravel these theories and to consider how they explain students' coping behaviour within the distance learning context.

The final chapter, *Chapter 6*, will draw together the theories and evidence presented in this book. This chapter will conclude with opportunities for readers to reflect on their own experiences of learning and how they developed coping strategies.

Reflection

Think about your own experience as a student:

- What competing demands have you had to negotiate?
- What coping strategies have you used?
- How closely do your coping strategies resemble theories of coping presented in this chapter?
- What can you learn from the three case studies in developing coping strategies for distance learning?

Practical activity

If you are studying as a distance learner, devise an action plan that takes into account your preferred approach to study and enables you to make the most of the resources at your disposal.

References

Abouserie R (1996) Stress, coping strategies and job satisfaction in university academic staff. *Educat Psychol* **16**(1): 49–56

Adejumo O, Brysiewicz P (1998) Coping strategies adopted by Baccalaureate nursing students in a problem-based learning programme. *Educ Health* **11**(3): 349–59

Bailey D, Moore J (1989) Closing the distance: Counselling at OU residential schools. *J Guid Counsel* **17**(3): 317–30

Carnwell R (1999) Distance education and the need for dialogue. *Open Learn* **14**(1): 50–5

Carnwell R, Moreland N, Helm R (2001) A comparison of the learning support needs of campus and distance based students. *Res Post-Compuls Educ* **6**: 1

Carver CS, Scheier MF, Weintraub JK (1989) Assessing coping strategies: a theoretically based approach. *J Personal Social Psychol* **56**: 267–83

Cohen F (1987) Measurement of Coping. In: Kasl SV, Cooper CL (eds). *Stress and Health: Issues in Research Methodology*. John Wiley & Sons, Chichester

Cohen F, Lazarus RS (1979) Coping with the stresses of illness. In: Stone GC, Cohen F, Adler NE, and assoc. *Health Psychology—A handbook: Theories, Applications, and Challenges of a Psychological Approach to the Health Care System*. Jossey-Bass, San Francisco: 217–54

Green CP (1987) Multiple role women: The real world of the mature RN learner. *J Nurs Educ* **26**(7): 266–71

Hargreaves D (1978) The significance of classroom coping strategies. In: Barton L, Meighan R (eds). *Sociological Interpretations of Schooling and Classroom: A Reappraisal*. Nafferton Books. Driffield: 73–100

Holahan CJ, Moos RH (1987) Personal and contextual determinants of coping strategies. *J Personal Social Psychol* **62**: 946–55

Kember D (1995) *Open Learning Courses for Adults: A Model of Student Progress*. Educational Technology Publications, New Jersey

Kirkup G, von Prummer C (1990) Support and connectedness: The needs of women distance education students. *J Dist Educ* **5**(2): 9–31

Knowles M (1980) How do you get people to become self-directed learners? *Train Devel J* **May**: 96–9

Lawton S (1997) Supportive learning in distance education. *J Adv Nurs* **25**: 1076–83

Lebel C (1989) Le support a l'etudiant en enseignement a distance. *J Dist Educ* **IV**(2): 7–24

Moreland N, Carnwell R (2000) Co-opting learners: Addressing their learning support needs through a learning support needs questionnaire. Part One: the rationale and basis of the learning support needs questionnaire. *Res Post-Compuls Educ* **5**(2): 173–91

Pascoe EJ (1977) For older college women. *McCalls* **March**

Pearlin LI Schooler C (1978) The structure of coping. *J Health Social Behav* **19**: 2–21

Peplau H (1952) *Interpersonal Relations in Nursing*. Macmillan Publishing, Basingstoke

Pym FR (1992) Women and distance education: A nursing perspective. *J Adv Nur* **17**: 383–9

Pym FR, Atkinson AM (1990) Reaching out via distance education to nurses: Needs assessment, planning and implications. Paper presented at the third congress of the Canadian Association for Distance Education, Quebec City. In: Pym FR (1992) Women and distance education: A nursing perspective. *J Adv Nurs* **17**: 383–9

Scheier MF, Carver CS (1977) Self-focused attention and the expression of emotion: Attraction, repulsion, elation, and depression. *J Personal Social Psychol* **35**: 625–36

Stark S, Warne T (1999) 'Connecting' the distance: Relational issues for participants in a distance learning programme. *J Furth High Educ* **23**(3): 391–402

Vowles B (1990) Educational guidance. *Conference Proceedings of Student Learning in the Open University—Process and Practice*. Open University Press, Milton Keynes

6
Organising your learning and moving forward

Introduction

This book began by discussing the characteristics, advantages and limitations of distance learning as a mode of study. These were compared with campus-based study in relation to the differing roles that tutors should adopt in their interactions with students. A case was made for distance learning being a valuable mode of study for women, since it offers flexibility for those wishing to continue full-time work at the same time as engaging in further study, in order to achieve academic credit.

Throughout the book, readers have been invited to apply theories and evidence to their own situation, an approach that is consistent with a distance learning philosophy. The characteristics and needs of women distance learners have also remained paramount throughout the text. *Chapter 2* focussed on learning styles, strategies and approaches to study, and activities were provided to assist personal application and reflection. *Chapters 3* and *4* focussed on the three approaches to study identified through interviews of twenty women distance learners. These approaches to study were considered in the light of student habits, such as selection of and commitment to reading, as well as student learning preferences. It was argued that these findings have important implications for curriculum design, including design of text materials, the role of tutors, and provision of guidance and support. Providing good quality support systems for students helps them to be organised and achieve higher level outcomes. Three concepts were, thus, proposed that reflect the distance learning process—need for guidance, approaches to studying, and engagement with materials. These concepts combine to influence the support needs and coping strategies that students adopt, this being the main focus of *Chapter 5*.

This final chapter encourages readers to reflect on the previous chapters in relation to their own career advancement. It enables them to consider whether distance learning is an appropriate method for their particular learning needs. Concluding activities encourage readers to consider their own particular style, strategy and approach to study, and how these translate into learning needs. Readers are invited to consider what coping strategies they need to adopt in order to progress through the learning process successfully.

Section one—is distance learning an appropriate method of learning?

The main characteristics of distance learning are included in *Table 1.1* of *Chapter 1*. These include: flexibility, autonomy, freedom for students to pursue their own goals, and active engagement in in-depth study. From the evidence presented throughout this book, however, these advantages need to be viewed with caution. Flexibility and autonomy can only exist within the constraints of the curriculum. Thus, materials have to be read and understood within a limited time period, and assessed work has to be completed. Nevertheless, distance learning does release students from the need to travel to distant locations at times that are inconvenient to them, except of course, for the regular evening tutorials, which often tend to be a feature of distance learning provision. Before considering whether distance learning is a worthwhile mode of study, it is worth also considering the limitations presented in *Table 1.1* of *Chapter 1*. These include the view of knowledge as a commodity, in that course writers decide what students should know. In class-based study, decisions about what students should know are (or should be) negotiated between tutors and students, through the medium of course materials.

Distance learning has also been accused of subordinating students' needs to the learning package, so that students become passive recipients of knowledge, which is often reflected in their regurgitation of materials in assessed work. The counter-argument to this, is that students can engage deeply with materials if they so wish. Furthermore, the extent to which they achieve this will be determined by their learning characteristics, such as learning style and approach to study, as well as the amount of support they are given. As for regurgitation of materials, campus-based students are just as likely to regurgitate the lecturer's point of view noted during a lecture, or the viewpoint of a particular author, as distance learners are likely to regurgitate distance learning materials.

Whether distance learning is an appropriate method of study is, therefore, a matter of personal choice. What became evident, during the research for this book, is that students are less likely to enjoy the learning experience if they have misconceptions of what distance learning is about and expect regular and close proximity with tutors. Students who gained most from distance learning had often prepared for study in advance and were motivated to learn from the experience itself, rather than merely to gain credits, so that they could gain access to a degree course. Such students had made appropriate arrangements for gaining support from their family and tended to be quite organised in arranging a timetable for study. Distance learning will always be a difficult option for some students, as their home circumstances will make so many competing demands upon them that, even with excellent support systems from the institution, the learning experience is likely to impose more strain than their resources are able to cope with. Such students will, therefore, need to develop clear coping strategies in advance, and this will be discussed later in this chapter.

Despite the importance of support and coping strategies, other learner characteristics also play a part in determining the success of distance learning. Before considering learning styles, strategies, and approaches to study, readers are invited to consider whether distance learning is likely to be an appropriate method of study, given their personal circumstances.

Reflection

- Bearing in mind the advantages and limitations of distance learning, is it compatible with your personal circumstances?
- Are your circumstances such that you would be able to find time and space to study at home without excessive interruptions?
- Would your reasons for studying by distance learning involve a determined choice because the philosophy appeals to you, or would it be the only method of studying available?

Actions needed

- Given your responses to the above questions, what actions, if any do you need to take to prepare yourself for distance learning study?

Section two—is your learning style, strategy or approach to study compatible with distance learning?

A variety of learning styles, strategies, approaches to study, and learning preferences have been discussed in this book, and approaches to study, in particular, have been researched in relation to distance learning. The definitions and distinctions between these terms are presented in *Table 2.1* in *Chapter 2*. The theories are discussed using Curry's (1983) analogy of an onion, with cognitive processes operating at the inner level, and learning preferences, being closer to the outside world, operating at the outer layer. The value of approaches to study is that, being towards the middle layer of the onion, they draw on the literature concerning learning styles and strategies, as well as being influenced by, and in turn influencing, learning preferences. The properties of the three approaches to study (see *Table 3.1* in *Chapter 3*), illustrate how the literature can be applied to each one.

Vermunt's (1996) style theory, for example, can be applied to all three approaches to study. Application-directed learners had some similarities with both speedy-focussers and global dippers, whereas systematic waders seemed to be more reproduction-directed. Systematic waders also bear some resemblance to Pask's (1976) serialist learner and Sternberg's (1990) executive function of self-government. Both the speedy-focusser and global dipper approaches can be also explained by Witkin *et al*'s (1977) theory of field dependence. The solitary nature of systematic waders makes them field independent, while the preference of global dippers to learn with other people makes them field dependent. Unlike the other two approaches, speedy-focussers seem to be impulsive learners (Kagan *et al*, 1964) as they reach decisions quickly after a brief review of opinions.

Learning preferences, discussed in *Chapter 2*, are also important to distance learning, since they indicate the most popular modes of study for different types of learners. Much of the research suggests that students prefer to work closely with tutors, to have lectures and demonstrations presented to them, and to have very specific assignment guidance. This combination suggests a preference for dependent, rather than independent learning. Although students might prefer these methods, this does not mean that dependent learning is in students' best interest. The most recent research into learning preferences was conducted by Sadler-Smith (1997), and suggests that dependent learners prefer teacher-directed, highly structured programmes, with explicit assignments set and assessed by the teacher. These students also prefer lectures and tutorial/surgeries. By comparison, collaborative learners prefer discussion, group assignments and social interaction, while independent learners prefer to exercise an influence on the content and structure of the learning programmes with the teacher as a resource (Sadler-Smith, 1997). Independent learners and, to a lesser extent, collaborative learners, are well-suited to distance learning.

It was noted in *Chapter 4* that the main significance of approaches to study is their impact upon curriculum design. This includes activities, such as designing distance learning packages, providing tutorials, and making other types of support and guidance accessible. *Table 4.9* in *Chapter 4* identifies the properties and dimensions of the three approaches to study. In attempting to meet the needs of the different types of student, distance learning materials should be designed in a manner that all students will engage with them sufficiently to achieve a deep level of learning. Tutorials should be provided for groups, as well as for individuals, both face-to-face and by telephone. Only in this way can the 'passive' tutor role be provided for some students and the 'active' tutor role for others. Other types of guidance include dialogue and support. Types of dialogue include that provided within the package for students whose learning style matches this approach, and with other people for students who learn through collaboration. Support was characterised as academic provided by the institution, as well as emotional support and practical support, both of which students might need to access from other sources.

Support was found to be an important feature of distance learning and this was addressed further in *Chapter 5* in relation to coping strategies. Before returning to the concepts of support and coping strategies, readers are invited to reflect on their learning styles, approaches to study and learning preferences, and their compatibility with distance learning.

Reflection

Return to the activity completed at the end of *Chapter 2*.

- How appropriate is your style, strategy, approach to learning and learning preferences, to distance learning?
- Are the alternatives, if any, that you decided achievable within the desired time scale?
- Given your personal learning characteristics, what would you expect from distance learning in terms of:
  - design of distance learning materials
  - the role of the tutor
  - support systems?

Actions needed

If you are considering distance learning as a mode of study, decide how you intend to find out whether the design of the course will meet your particular needs.

Section three—support needs and the development of coping strategies

The main focus of *Chapter 5* was on support and coping strategies for distance learners. Support was viewed as a means of enabling students to *connect* with the learning process, as well as with tutors and students.

The concept of 'connectedness' was discussed drawing on recent studies, such as Lawton (1997) and Stark and Warne (1999). These authors stressed the nature of the student/tutor relationship and continuity, as well as the need to provide structure and guidance within this relationship. Both authors draw on concepts of counselling to inform their work. This is an interesting concept and indicates the way in which the distance learning process might differ significantly from class-based study. This is also implicit within students' need to develop coping strategies.

The concept of coping strategies also formed an important component of *Chapter 5*. Theories of coping emerge from psychological, as well as sociological literature. Attempts have been made by psychologists to measure coping strategies, although there seems to be general agreement that measurement of the phenomenon of coping is difficult. Since most people draw on resources around them, as well as their own personality characteristics, in attempting to cope with strainful situations, theories of sociology become important in understanding coping. Understanding how people cope, mirrors attempts to understand people's learning styles, in that we need to understand cognitive (thinking) variables, as well as how people respond to their world. Curry's (1983) Onion Model (see *Chapter 2*) could be used to understand people's coping strategies, as well as their learning styles, strategies, approaches, and preferences. Curry's Onion Model has, therefore, been adapted to incorporate learning style theory, as well as learning support needs and coping strategies (*Figure 6.1*).

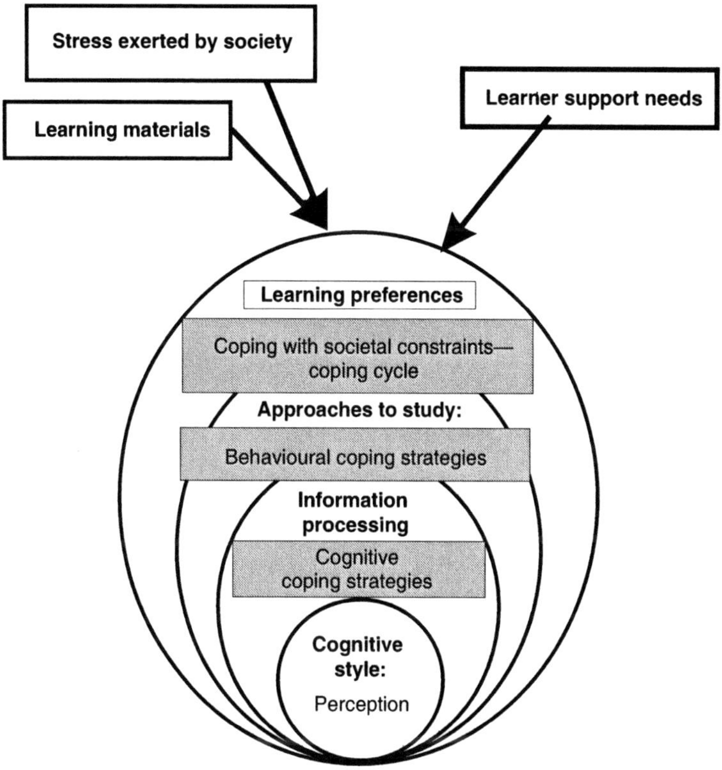

Figure 6.1: An adaptation of Curry's Onion Model to include coping strategies

At the inner layer of the model, cognitive learning style, i.e. the way in which people think about their learning, corresponds to the way in which they think about and perceive stressful events. At this level, this might explain why some students adopt certain learning styles and have perceptions about stressful events that allow them to progress through learning experiences without difficulty. At the next layer of the onion, students use information processing such as Kolb's learning cycle. Corresponding to this, is the way in which students use their inner resources, such as self-confidence, as well as problem-focussed and emotion-focussed coping strategies. Problem-focussed strategies (Adejumo and Brysiewicz, 1998) include: increasing effort, putting aside other things that prevent them getting on with academic work, and pausing to consider how to deal with their workload. Emotion-focussed strategies include: positive re-interpretation (i.e., using inner resources to try to see the positive side of the stressful experience), accepting the situation, or using denial. These coping strategies are within the inner layer of the onion because they do not rely on other people. Coping strategies associated with the outer layers of the onion, however, begin to rely on other resources outside of the individual and to affect other people.

Moving towards the outer layer of the onion, problem-focussed strategies might involve asking other people for advice on the assignment, or dysfunctional strategies of behaviourally disengaging from the learning experience (i.e. giving up), or mentally disengaging by immersion in other activities (which might or might not involve other people), as a distraction from the stress. Alcohol or drug disengagement might also occur at this level and is also likely to affect, or be affected by, other people. At the outer level of the onion, learning preferences become important, and these preferences, if met, might become part of students' coping strategies. Coping strategies here might include seeking advice and reassurance from tutors and other students, as well as the emotion-focussed strategy of venting emotions.

Conclusion

Approaches to study, and their impact on support and guidance needs, have been discussed throughout this text and evidence has been sought from the literature, as well as empirical research. The book has concluded with the importance of coping strategies as a mechanism by which students can be proactive in gaining the support they need. The book would not be complete without a final opportunity to reflect on this evidence, as it applies to distance learning. A final reflective activity, therefore, follows.

Reflection

- How important is support to you as a means of connecting with the learning experience?
- Which of the three types of support, if any, is most important to you?
- How successful have you been in gaining access to the support you need?
- Refer back to the reflective activity at the end of chapter five
- If you have decided to embark on a distance learning programme, what coping strategies do you need to consider developing to prepare you for the learning experience?

References

Adejumo O, Brysiewicz P (1998) Coping strategies adopted by Baccalaureate nursing students in a problem-based learning programme. *Educ Health* **11**(3): 349–59

Curry L (1983) An organisation of learning styles and theory constructs. *ERIC document* **235**: 185

Kagan J, Rosman BL, Day D, Albert J, Philips W (1964) Information processing in the child: Significance of analytic and reflective attitudes. *Psycholog Mon* **78**: 1

Lawton S (1997) Supportive learning in distance education. *J Adv Nurs* **25**: 1076–83

Pask G (1976) Styles and strategies of learning. *Br J Educat Psychol* **46**: 128–48

Sadler-Smith E (1997) 'Learning style': Frameworks and instruments. *Educat Psychol* **17**(1and2): 51–63

Stark S, Warne T (1999) 'Connecting' the distance: Relational issues for participants in a distance learning programme. *J Furth High Educ* **23**(3): 391–402

Sternberg RJ (1990) Thinking styles: Keys to understanding human performance. *Phi Delta Kappan* **71**: 366–71

Vermunt JD (1996) Metacognitive, cognitive and affective aspects of learning styles and strategies: A phenomenographic analysis. *High Educ* **31**: 25–50

Witkin HA, Moore C, Goodenough D, Cox P (1977) Field-dependent and field-independent cognitive styles and their educational implications. *Rev Educat Res* **47**: 1–64

Index

S

T

V